THE GIANT AT MY BACK

A YEAR LIVING IN
THE SHADOW OF DEMENTIA

Carolyn Donnelly

First published in Great Britain in 2021

Instant Apostle
104 The Drive
Rickmansworth
Herts
WD3 4DU

if notified, will formally seek permission at the earliest opportunity.

British Library Cataloguing-in-Publication Data

A catalogue record for this book is available from the British Library.

This book and all other Instant Apostle books are available from Instant Apostle:

Website: www.instantapostle.com

Email: info@instantapostle.com

ISBN 978-1-912726-43-1

Printed in Great Britain.

For Ralph

Contents

Contents

Introduction

In the late nineteenth century, infectious diseases were the major cause of morbidity and mortality for both men and women, for young and old alike. As decades passed, thanks to the introduction of childhood vaccinations, the provision of clean water and cleaner air along with significant public health legislation on housing, environment and nutrition, they began to wane. Scientific advances and an emerging understanding of how to treat and cure some of these diseases also contributed to their decline. However, having been waiting in the wings, other conditions such as heart diseases, cancers and strokes began to emerge and exert their impact on the morbidity and mortality statistics of the nation.

Thanks to focused and persistent efforts in the twentieth century to tackle some of these conditions, death rates for heart disease and stroke have halved for both men and women in the United Kingdom since 2001 and survival rates for a number of cancers have improved greatly. Inevitably, though, as these conditions have lessened their grip on the ill-health of the population, another quiver of diseases has stepped into their leading position. Since 2001, deaths from dementia and

Alzheimer's disease have increased by 60 per cent in men and doubled in women.[1]

Dementia can be described as a range of conditions that affect the brain health of individuals. People with dementia see their ability to think, remember and learn decrease over time, and may also have problems with communication and experience disorientation or delusions. They can display changes in their mood, behaviour and personality. Dementia mostly, but not exclusively, affects people aged over sixty, and after the age of sixty-five the prevalence of dementia has been shown to double with each additional five years of life. More than half of all dementias are attributed to Alzheimer's disease, with one-fifth caused by vascular dementia.[2] The diagnosis of mixed dementia, a mixture of both Alzheimer's and vascular dementia, is also common. It is estimated that there are currently 23,735 people in Northern Ireland living with dementia and that this figure is likely to rise to 57,500 by 2051.[3]

---

[1] Public Health England, 'Health Profile for England: 2017' (July 2017), pp 3-4, www.gov.uk/government/publications/health-profile-for-england/chapter-2-major-causes-of-death-and-how-they-have-changed (accessed 7th August 2020).
[2] Department of Health, Social Services and Public Safety, 'Improving dementia services in Northern Ireland – a regional strategy' (November 2011), www.health-ni.gov.uk/publications/improving-dementia-services-northern-ireland-regional-strategy (accessed 1st January 2021).
[3] HSC Public Health Agency, 'Director of Public Health Annual Report 2018' (October 2019), pp 28-29,

But in the end, regardless of what it is called or sub-diagnosed as and whatever symptoms it displays in individuals, dementia is a disease or condition that affects people. It affects you and me. Like other progressive degenerative conditions, it is not only the individual who has the diagnosis who is impacted by it. Dementia affects families, especially the wife, husband, partner, children and friends of those with the condition, and in no small way it also has an impact on society as a whole.

In spring 2017, dementia came to our home when my husband, Ralph, was diagnosed with the condition. We were just about to celebrate our twenty-sixth wedding anniversary, and while the diagnosis was not unexpected, it still came as a tremendous shock to me. Our life as we knew it was going to change forever with his diagnosis and I knew that, as his wife, I would have to be the overseer of that change. Sadly, by that stage Ralph was incapable of even knowing change was happening, let alone actively managing it.

I had taken early retirement from a career in the health service in Northern Ireland in March 2015, as by that stage his health had deteriorated to the point where he could not be left by himself and I knew that I needed to be with him full-time. When I had been planning my retirement during the last years that I worked, I had hoped that Ralph and I would have many good years together; that we could travel to new countries, or even just see more of our own, and share lots of new experiences. However, with his

www.publichealth.hscni.net/publications/director-public-health-annual-report-2018 (accessed 1st January 2021).

diagnosis and rapidly deteriorating mental and physical health, sadly that was not to be.

This book describes the first year of our changed life following Ralph's diagnosis of mixed dementia and how I tried to cope with all that that entailed for me, as of necessity I had to become his full-time carer. I describe it as a journey. Our dementia journey, or 'D' journey as I came to call it. Ralph and I set out on it together without knowing where it would take us or how we would live through it day by day, but having set out on it, the only thing I knew for certain was that there was no possibility of turning back.

Did we have a typical first year journey for this diagnosis? Who knows? It was our journey and as such was unique, special and precious to us. Did we travel it well? Again, who knows? Especially not me. However, having set out on the first year of our dementia journey, Ralph and I laughed and cried separately and together on it, and throughout it experienced and learned so much about ourselves, each other and other people.

But as I, the chronicler of this journey, look back over this first year, most of all I have realised how much I have learned and experienced about God in and through this time. I came to accept that while this is a journey that neither Ralph nor I would willingly have chosen to set out on, one year later, I – and, I hope, he if he were able to – could say it is one through which we have been incredibly blessed and enriched.

Author's note: I am not a theologian and have no formal biblical study qualifications. I am simply a Christian who loves God's

Word and daily looks to it for guidance, strength, encouragement and, at times, chastening and correction. My interpretations and views on the Bible passages I use throughout the book are entirely my own, and if theologically incorrect, the error is mine alone. They are shared as thoughts and reflections that came to me at that particular time in Ralph's and my 'D' journey and helped and supported me through it.

1
Our Dementia Journey Begins

Why is it that so often we give places names or titles that are the very antithesis of the function that the place in question is known for or provides? Take the name 'health centre', for example. Was there ever a less apt name? Surely the main reason for going to a health centre is because at the very least you feel less than healthy and at the very most you feel the exact opposite of it. Perhaps it is a classic example of how, as a society, we always tend to accentuate the positive at the expense of being honest about the reality.

Sitting in a such-named health facility in our local town, I was struck by the herculean efforts the health care providers of this centre had made in their interior design approach to mask the reality of its function. Gone were the clinical white walls and institutional hard chairs that scraped across polished concrete floors of such places in the last century. In their place, there were soft individual seats of various heights and sizes, covered in complementary colours of soft heather and green fabrics that sat against pale lemon and sky-blue walls, grounded by office-quality durable carpet tiles. Gone also were the garish posters that would have adorned those walls in previous decades, proclaiming to all who had the misfortune to be waiting for whatever health – or more aptly, sickness – care was their allotted portion that day. They illustrated the benefits of healthy eating, gave dire warnings or even apportioned blame for not washing your hands after having been to the toilet… and then, of course, there were those special ones. Discreetly tucked away in one corner, they often, in allegory or even in cartoon fashion, issued even starker warnings about the risk of sexually transmitted diseases. No, now the walls were, for the most part, clear of any adornment at all, save a carefully positioned framed print of a sailboat heading out into a vast, still ocean, and an abstract print of a vase of flowers beside which sat a pot of tea and two cups and saucers. All the place needed was a plate of bourbons on the ubiquitous square occasional table sandwiched between two chairs at a corner of the waiting area and we could nearly all join in the required illusion of health and normality, if not utilitarianism and boredom.

But of course, the reality was far from the wannabe picture suggested by this waiting area. The only reason any of us were sitting in this politically correct, décor-neutral and background music-free space was the flip side of the façade presented. It was because we were there to be told, or for some to be told more, about the impact of the lack of health in our own or our loved ones' lives. For me, it was finally to face the fear that had been creeping up on me for the last months and even years, if I were honest. It was to meet the giant that had been waiting in the background of our lives; to look him square in the eyes and bow beneath the enormity of his presence, and to finally come to a place in my life where I would have to accept that he would now be ever present in our future.

Our first appointment

As I sat there on that warm sunny March morning in 2017, the enormity of what our date with destiny here would bring lay heavily on my shoulders. I looked around at the others waiting there like us, and saw in some of them what that destiny might look like. For the most part, people were sitting in pairs, some of similar ages to Ralph, whom I took to be couples, and others more likely to be an ageing parent and child combination. One of the pair was, in the main, reasonably to very well dressed; the men in coordinating shirt and jumper and the women similarly colour matched, perhaps with a necklace to complement the outfit – possibly a special birthday or even a wedding present that was undoubtedly aired on all special occasions, of which this definitely qualified as one. Today, however, the necklace was worn underneath a gaping collar that evidenced a thinner and more wrinkled neck than at the time of the gift or purchase. Then, of course, for both genders, there were good, solid shoes. The sort you would never have been seen dead in at the height of youthfulness, but now of necessity providing both safety for shuffling feet and security for the one sitting beside them.

That person was, in this setting, now labelled the carer. The one who provided that steadying arm for, or hand on the back of, the client, as we now had to refer to the patient, as they steered their rollator or Zimmer frame through life. This person, the carer, unlike their partner, the client, was frazzled and uncoordinated and had the appearance of living life in a constant rush. They wore a hastily donned jacket or coat, hiding wrinkled sleeves of a shirt or blouse, as an unexpected toilet run had been required by the person they now sat beside before leaving for this not-to-be missed appointment, meaning that there was no time to check appearances in a mirror, let alone go to the spare room to get the sports jacket or coat that would have been the preferred dress in which to attend the doctor's appointment. In my case, it meant no lip gloss, and grabbing the first coat that my hand connected with in the cloakroom, which signalled to all that I was expecting a downpour and was ready for it in my full-length waterproof.

As I sat there looking at the other people around us, who also sat quietly waiting in this place we had all been summoned to, I wondered what they saw when they looked at Ralph and me sitting opposite or alongside them. We were definitely a couple, as I sat there holding Ralph's hand while we waited to be called, and occasionally he would look at me and smile his beautiful smile. We had always held hands, even from the first time we went out together.

Amazingly, that was virtually a blind date. Ralph had got my phone number from a friend, phoned me and, to my great surprise, asked me out for a meal. I was in my early thirties and single. I was happy in my career in the health service in Northern Ireland and had absolutely no thought of considering looking for a boyfriend, let alone a husband. I was content to be single and had no expectation that that would ever change. As I was to discover on that first date, Ralph was a widower with five grown-up children and four grandchildren, but that didn't concern me any more than the obvious age gap between us. What did concern me on that first date was whether he had a Christian faith, as I couldn't contemplate a relationship with any man if he were not a Christian. Fortunately, it didn't take long on our car journey to the restaurant where he had booked a table, for both of us to find out, through some subtle questions to each other, that, as we would say in Northern Ireland, we were both 'well saved'. Ralph had committed his life to Christ in his early twenties and had continued to attend Brethren Assembly meetings in Gospel Halls. I was from a Methodist family and had committed my life to Christ as a young child. Our shared faith was the rock on which our relationship began and continued to be the foundation of our life together.

In the middle of my musings, while I tried to ready myself for the meeting with the doctor, Ralph was blissfully unaware of the significance of this appointment. We could have been in a coffee shop or our local shopping centre for all he knew, and probably that is where he did think we were, as it was his default for when I said we were going out. As long as I was there, Ralph's world was safe and secure. He just got in the car when I said we were going out, and sat quietly until I took us to where we were appointed to be on this or any morning.

I spoke quietly to him to say we were early for our appointment and we would just wait until we were called.

He just smiled back and held my hand. It struck me then that his life would be like this from now on. Waiting. Waiting for appointments, waiting for me and on me to be with him. In the quiet that was the waiting area, apart from the usual comings and goings of such a place, I had a sudden frightening thought that perhaps he was in fact waiting to die, but I quickly put that out of my mind. I told myself firmly that we were both waiting together to see what the next phase of our living would be like.

As time flicked by on the digital clock on the wall – another sign of the times that the healthy silence was not even interrupted by the ticking of a clock – individuals and couples shuffled or sped up and down the adjoining corridor. It was not hard to recognise the professionals with their purposeful walk, heads bowed and arms full of papers and files going in and out of rooms without knocking or asking, and equally not hard to identify the others – the ones here to be seen. The patiently waiting, the problems, the case studies, and then the newbies like us. We were the clean, pristine slim files, yet to be filled with reports of assessments by a range of professionals we had still to meet; files that would be filled with the results of blood tests and scans and myriads of copy letters to GPs and other interested parties, all of which would be circulated widely to everyone but us.

Eventually our turn came, or rather Ralph's turn, as I was to be sidelined initially while he was taken away by a nurse. I was advised I would be called to see the doctor later. Even though we were in this special place, where Ralph and others like him received special care and attention by professional individuals specially trained to provide it, I worried for him and about him, as he was now alone, with strangers and without me; that is when I really began to consider the enormity of why we were here; the reality of what this hour in this place would mean and what our lives would become. Because here Ralph would get his label, his diagnosis, his destiny, and it would be that most fearful of all labels, to me even more fearful than the cancer label. It would be that cancer of the mind: dementia. Oh, he would get a definitive label, I knew. It would have a clinical subtitle, an unspellable name, but it would be his destiny and, by covenant, my calling. Ralph would have the dementia and Carolyn would have the working out of it; a skewed partnership, where the greater would become the lesser, the leader the led and the provider the receiver. We would for his evermore be defined as the cared for and the carer, and wait together for others and each other in the shrinking world that would become our lives.

Ralph's diagnosis

Eventually it was my turn to be shown in to see the doctor, who looked more like an A-level student than a doctor well on the way to being a consultant; to sit in a smaller version of the waiting area and look into the eyes of a much younger woman who had spent all of her morning looking into the eyes of people like I had now become. A carer, a person to be contacted, spoken to and with about the cared for. Someone who in essence would take over Ralph's life, would speak for him, stand up for him, protect him from others and himself and, in turn, be defined by my connection to him. As I sat and listened, she outlined what she had asked Ralph in terms of questions posed time and time again in initial and repeat appointments in this place. I learned from what she said to me that there had been a significant deterioration since he had been seen in the assessment clinic three months earlier.

And at last, from this doctor I had never met and might never meet again, I heard the label's name. Actually, two names, as I was to discover. For Ralph, the double challenge of having mixed dementia (Alzheimer's disease and vascular dementia). A double portion of confusion. Two parallel lines of decay travelling at different rates but ultimately reaching the same destination. We were now officially diagnosed, defined and dispatched on the dementia journey; a well-travelled if meandering path that would take us both to places that we never would have willingly or intentionally sought and which would ultimately lead Ralph away from me into his own unique world. The file in front of her would begin to be filled up and grow fatter with papers all about him, and various files with his name would now be opened in several offices across the service providers we would interact with in the future. We would be in filing cabinets and spreadsheets, on contact lists and desktop computers, and our personal details would now become shared property. Shared with people we would never meet and never know.

The giant was now unleashed and in the room. As I listened to the doctor go through what she and the team had planned in terms of future tests and appointments, I had an oppressive feeling of a heavy weight bearing down on my shoulders. She talked and I did listen, but I could not recall later any detail of what she said. I heard words like 'medication' and 'therapies', 'stimulation' and 'maintenance' and felt numbed by it all. I only felt an overpowering dread that this weight would get heavier and heavier in the coming days, weeks and months.

All this time Ralph was in another room, waiting for me to join him. The doctor said with a smile that he hadn't wanted to go back up to the waiting area but wanted me to come to him. I was really pleased to hear that. In some sad way it justified my presence with the doctor and my status with the system I was all too aware I was now entering. As if on cue, she then changed tack entirely and started to talk to me about me and my needs – as a wife, a carer, a point of contact, an enduring power of attorney. We talked about practicalities, about legalities, about services and support. In a clinical and logical way, we agreed some processes and timelines for Ralph and for me.

We were in and running. The system would now overtake us, if not take us over, and I had a flashback to something a young person had once said to me many years before when I asked them about their experience of health services. They said they felt that services had an opinion about them without even knowing them; they felt they were just a file passed round offices. I hoped that decades later, my experiences would be more positive. After all, this was a health centre and well-being was the name of the game we were all playing.

As we left the health centre, the sun was shining. It was such a beautiful spring day with trees in leaf. We could see some flowers with their happy colours of yellows and purples brightening up the roadside. As Ralph and I walked slowly back to the car, it was lovely to feel the gentle breeze on my face and sense the weak sun trying to warm what was a cool morning. I felt encouraged and calmed by the fact that what had been, to some extent, an unpleasant experience was ending with a memory of a bright and beautiful spring day.

Ralph was tired after all the walking up and down corridors and having people ask him interminable questions, so I got him into the car and told him we were going home. I had planned to take him for a cup of coffee after the appointment, but it was all a bit too overwhelming for me, let alone what he might be feeling. I just wanted to get us both back to the safety and sanctuary of our home.

As we drove, I asked Ralph what the doctor had said to him. He thought for a moment and then said that she had just asked him a lot of questions. I asked if he had been able to answer them. He just looked out of the car window and was quiet.

I debated with myself long and hard as to whether I would talk with Ralph about the diagnosis and what it was all likely to mean, and decided I would. As was the ability of his understanding so must be the level of our discussion, and as both were on a downward trajectory, it was either now or never.

Later that night, I asked him if he knew what the doctor had said was the matter with him, and he replied, 'No, not really.' So I told him that the doctor had said his forgetfulness was caused by dementia and that she had diagnosed that he had both Alzheimer's disease and vascular dementia and that he was going to get new tablets for it, and we would go back and see her in a few weeks. He just said, 'Oh.' Then he said he was tired, so the both of us lay down, side by side, on the bed and were quiet.

Dementia – my giant

When I was a child, church and Sunday school were a central part of my life. I was raised on Bible stories, parables and prophets, sin and redemption, failure and forgiveness. I particularly remember the Old Testament stories we were taught. The fall in the Garden of Eden; the almost-sacrifice of Isaac; Joseph's coat of many colours; the battles and victories; Samson and his long hair; the love story that was Ruth; Esther's wooing of a king to save her people and, of course, the forty-year wanderings the children of Israel had to endure in the desert because of their disobedience. They all faced their giants: literal ones, like David with Goliath, or perceived ones, like Moses, an unwilling leader. Yet they all overcame them. How? By an absolute belief that God was bigger than the giants that were in front of them, and by their living out of that belief in the actions they took. They accepted that while without God they could only see giants, with Him they were enabled to see that these giants were actually just mini characters in God's plan for their and their nation's lives. They came to realise that those giants would or could never prevent or stand in the way of them achieving God's will.

I realised that night that Ralph's dementia was my giant, both literal and metaphorical. Over the previous months it had been this looming presence in my life, influencing my thinking and actions. I knew that just like those Old Testament heroes and heroines, I needed to accept that I could never defeat this giant by myself, but I most certainly could vanquish its hold over me with God on my side. I determined not to try to hide from this giant of Ralph's dementia so that it was always at my back, lurking and hovering. Rather, I would keep it where I could see it. Face it and have it face me. I didn't know how I was going to do that, but I had an unswerving feeling that God knew, and as long as He did, Ralph and I would be alright. I determined that from now on, Ralph and I would use the 'D' word in conversation. That we would accept his forgetfulness and decreasing awareness of what was happening in and around him, and we would endeavour to live every moment of every day as best we could. I drew great encouragement from words that Paul wrote to the church at Philippi:

> I know what it is to be in need, and I know what it is to have plenty. I have learned the secret of being content in any and every situation, whether well fed or hungry, whether living in plenty or in want. I can do all this through him who gives me strength.
> *Philippians 4:12-13*

We would face this giant together. The three of us: Ralph, Carolyn and God. I prayed that wherever this journey would take us, Ralph and I would be given grace to find contentment where we were and strength to live each day, even in this new unknown, uncertain world of dementia.

2
Look Forward

I have had a blessed life. I was born into a Christian farming family, taught right and wrong, shown the importance of duty and respect and encouraged to study and work hard to earn rewards. As the psalmist records, 'The boundary lines have fallen for me in pleasant places; surely I have a delightful inheritance' (Psalm 16:6).

Or perhaps that is my take on it now, with the benefit of hindsight, a wonderful blessing in itself. Having to face the death of a parent at an early age, the disappointment of being turned down for the first career I thought would suit me and discovering three years into a four-year course that I really didn't like the career path that I had chosen, are also memories I recall from time to time. When I was diagnosed with thyroid cancer in 2002, I was particularly aggrieved and went through a brief phase of feeling very sorry for myself. Then in a wave of divine inspiration, I decided to write a list of the ten worst things that had happened to me up until that point in my life. Being diagnosed with cancer ranked fourth. Now, it would be much nearer tenth.

The day I married Ralph was undoubtedly the happiest day of my life, and on a list of the ten best things that ever happened to me it will always be number one. Marriage was so unexpected for me. When it passed me by in my twenties, I had come to the point where I had accepted that I was going to be single and, as I said before, I was content in that. So when Ralph came along, I was totally shocked at how quickly and completely I fell in love with him. Three weeks after we met, he asked me to marry him, and I said yes with absolutely no hesitation. We were married eight months to the day after we had our first meal out together.

Second marriages are challenging, regardless of the circumstances under which they take place. My mother died when I was young and my father then married Elizabeth, who became my best friend and confidante. More than that, unknown to me during those years, she would be my role model for my new place in Ralph's life and in that of his family. Elizabeth never tried to be a mother, stepmother or, when my siblings' children came along, a step-grandmother. She was just always Elizabeth. Never defined by what she was – a second wife, or a step-person – but rather defined by who she was, simply Elizabeth. That was what I wanted for me as I started a new life as part of Ralph's family in 1991 when we married. I wanted to be accepted for who I was and not for what I had become in his or their lives.

Understandably there were adjustments to be made by us all. Ralph had to accept that I was different from what his concept of what a wife was. I had to get used to someone else in my life 24/7 and his family had to come to terms with me now being in their dad's life. A special blessing to me in my new life were the grandchildren. Ralph was always called Pop by his grandchildren and to them I became, and have always been, simply Carolyn. Over the years, a total of fourteen grandchildren became and still are a central part of our shared lives and, to them, we were and always are just Pop and Carolyn.

Sharing the diagnosis with others

It was so hard to tell people of his diagnosis. I looked at the telephone for ages before I could pick it up to call everyone I wanted to share the news with. Ralph's children and my family all knew that something had been slowly going wrong for months. Thankfully, at least he and I had hidden the years that he had been slowly deteriorating from them. But to now have to repeatedly go over what the doctor had said and use words we had all been avoiding for so long was difficult. It was the word 'dementia'. Everyone had their own understanding of what that meant. Not always, perhaps, based on scientific fact, but more frequently on coffee conversations at work or gleaned from television programmes or newspaper articles skimmed over in years past.

There were tears and silences from his children, understanding words from an older generation who had personal experience of dementia in their own or extended family, and sad looks from those I spoke to in person, perhaps more for me than for Ralph. People offered me their advice and support, kind words and hugs and promises of practical help if and when it should be required. To have to tell the story and relive the diagnosis experience time and time again was exhausting, but finally I felt that everyone who needed to know did know and, most importantly, they had heard it from me.

The days following Ralph's diagnosis passed into weeks and took on an increasingly predictable pattern. I had been advised that routine was good for dementia patients, or rather for individuals living with dementia, as I now understood was the preferred terminology to use, and so routine was what we lived by. We went out to the same places on the same days of the week. We got up, showered, had meals and went to bed like we were in a military institution. If we were having coffee in our local Christian bookshop, it must be Tuesday morning. Inevitably I carried this routine into my own life and that of the house. Washing, cleaning and shopping were all carefully scheduled to fit into Ralph's routine, which was now our life's routine. Our lives were planned, organised and timetabled with precision, and I found myself waking up each morning with a sense that each day was to be marched, not ambled or sauntered, through. I went to bed each night with a sense of achievement if we had managed to keep to our planned routine for that day.

In the beginning, these routine days were interspersed with dementia-related appointments or visits to our house. We saw doctors, social workers, physiotherapists and, a new one to me, a representative of a navigator service (a service that pointed users to other services or organisations that might help to meet some of their needs). I had to clear out a drawer for the plethora of information and options presented to us in leaflet and clear folder format. While Ralph sat in his chair and smiled beautifully at anyone who called or whom we visited in their office, I took charge of contact lists and options for both the cared for and the carer.

I completed long forms about my needs. I learned that I could take courses in caring and that both of us could even avail ourselves of opportunities to meet others in the same situation. I also learned that, when the time came, whatever and whenever that time was, there was a variety of services that were available and appeared to me to be queuing up to support us. I was stunned with the level of support available, and enormously thankful that I lived in a country where such practical, emotional and financial support was the norm for people in our situation and with his diagnosis.

But to be perfectly honest, it was all a bit much.

Was it selfish of me not to want to share Ralph until I absolutely had to? Every day a little more of him dripped away and I didn't want to miss a second of the time that signified the last vestiges of our relationship. Ralph had always been an intensely private person, particularly about his body. He would hardly ever let me see him in any stage of undress, and we had always had an agreed rule that bathrooms were single-occupancy spaces. I was determined that I would care for him physically and practically by myself for as long as absolutely possible.

Gradually the appointments and calls lessened as we settled into the system and we eventually reached the point where contact with the services was at our discretion. Bliss. It was just us now.

An unsettling time

While Ralph settled down into a very quiet and peaceful routine, characterised by long periods of sleep each day, by contrast, I grew more unsettled. I found myself cleaning an already clean house. I devoured books of any genre. I reread books from my schooldays that I had discovered in the loft while cleaning up there as everywhere else had been thrice cleaned. I dabbled in writing down my feelings. Not daring to call this poetry, I referred to it in my mind as 'scribbling'. I poured out my feelings about this 'D' situation on to my tablet when I had a spare minute, then when I read it, deleted most of it as I was so ashamed of the feelings I had admitted. I wrote anger and grief. I wrote frustration and bitterness and, most shaming of all, I wrote about life after dementia – when I would get my life back.

Then I stopped writing because I thought it was too negative. I bought myself a 'teach yourself French' course and began to wrestle with verb tenses and grammatical constructs in a language that I had learned decades before. I invested in a variety of cookbooks and expanded our repertoire of meals. Then I bought a Pilates DVD and started to stretch muscles I didn't know I had, as I thought all this reflection and cooking was not healthy.

All the while, Ralph slept on. He could sleep for hours during the day, as well as all night. To me it was too much, but despite medication reviews and mentioning it at all our dwindling dementia appointments, it seemed just to be the way it was. I found it fascinating that all the professionals I discussed it with, with a sort of 'knowing' look often said I should be glad of this because at least he wasn't agitated or belligerent. I was aware that some people with dementia developed these traits, and I appreciated that I was fortunate that Ralph did not display aggression or anger towards me or others. But I couldn't be happy that he was sleeping his life away.

As time slipped by, my frenetic activity around the house also slowed down. As Ralph slept morning and afternoon, I lay on the top of the bed beside him and thought about all the things I should be doing but could see no point in starting. As he started to mutter in his sleep, and at times startle himself into wakefulness shouting out things that had obviously just come into his mind, like, 'Where are the children?' 'Why are the accounts not done?' 'When are we going home?' 'I don't like this place!', I grew quieter. It seemed pointless to clean or cook healthy meals. I lowered my standards and bought easy meals and pre-prepared vegetables and potatoes. We increasingly ate pasta and rice as this didn't require peeling or scraping. I couldn't see the reason for showering every day as I didn't do enough to create any sweat. I let my hair grow out and ignored his daughters' comments that I was beginning to lose interest in myself.

I began, in my mind, to relive the life that I used to have and that I had revelled in. I had been gainfully employed up to the point when I had had to take early retirement to look after Ralph, and while I never even considered doing anything else, I began to reflect on what I had lost. A busy responsible job. Taking meetings, taking decisions, managing staff, oversight of a budget. I wondered where I would have reached in my career. I had ended my career at the level of middle management. Would I ever have made the final tier and reached top management? Would I have sought other promotion opportunities in my then, or in another, organisation? People used to know my name, I signed letters, I took important phone calls; and now I just did the dishes, I mopped up accidents, I collected his pension. I was now only Ralph's wife, his carer, his chauffeur and his maid. I felt I shouldn't be feeling like this, but I couldn't help it. I realised that I was insignificant and anonymous to the real world. I was invisible and becoming more so. I worried about my own mortality and who would take care of Ralph if anything were to happen to me. I worried about myself, about who would look after me. I wrote lists of instructions in the event of my death and told others where to find them. I completed my own power of attorney forms in case I succumbed to a life-limiting condition and couldn't take care of our affairs.

When I had done and completed every single thing I could think of, I finally admitted my grief at the state of my life, and I cried. I cried for a lost love and a curtailed life. I cried for all the places we talked about but would never visit. I cried for the times we had had and the times that we would never have. I cried that I was no longer a wife but a carer. I cried for Ralph and I cried for me. And when I had no more tears, I was just quiet and lay beside him on the top of our bed and contemplated the stillness that was now our life at this time in our 'D' journey.

Thankfully, it was in that stillness, which I gradually came to see as a welcome part of my now life, that I realised something. Despite how hard I pretended or tried,

I wasn't content in the situation I now found myself and Ralph in. In fact, I was anything but content. I was angry, I was disappointed, I was regretful and I was resentful. Sadly, most of all, I had to accept that I was a hypocrite because I tried so hard in front of everyone else to be the dutiful wife, the caring carer, the life organiser and the all-round good egg when in actual fact inside I was becoming a bitter, twisted old woman. The sham life I was trying to lead was eating away inside me and leaving a person I neither liked nor respected, so how would anyone else ever like or respect me? Not only was this 'D' life we were now both forced to live taking Ralph away from me, it was also taking me away from me.

I was letting the giant get behind me, letting him poke me with his long, gnarled fingers of envy and grief for the life I had lost and allowing his web of lethargy and apathy to pull me down. I reluctantly had to admit to myself that it was actually me who had put the giant behind me and that the very fact of doing that meant I had to look back. I was looking back at my work life and at my marital life, and looking back at times when Ralph and I had both been active and busy together. I was looking back at the life we had before our 'D' life of now. And the result of this looking back? I was totally and hopelessly dissatisfied with where I was and where I thought I was inevitably heading to. I was grieving for where I had come from and the life I'd had. Like those traipsing children of Israel, I longed for what I saw as the better times of the past. I forgot the pressures of work that I had succumbed to in those latter years of my working life. The long days, the extra hours, the rushed times with Ralph that were all I could give in those last hectic years. The nights when I couldn't sleep for worrying about my work. The constant sense that I wasn't good enough for my job and that I had to work harder and longer than my colleagues just to keep up with them. I saw only roses and good times when in fact there had been lots of thorns and difficult times too.

Lot's wife looked back

I thought of Lot's wife, in Genesis 19; a woman with no name who is only defined by her relationship to her husband and whom we are commanded to remember only because she looked back. I have often wondered: is she a victim of bad Christian press? After all, she had married Lot and spent years wandering the desert with him, living as a nomad in tents that were moved to follow the grazing for the sheep. Having to give birth to and raise her daughters on the hoof. Then at last, I'm sure to her great delight, finally settling in a city and setting up a home that was permanent. I'm sure, given Lot's status as a wealthy herdsman, she had a fine house on a good street and neighbours that she entertained or was entertained by. People would have known her name, she would have had servants to manage and a household to oversee.

Then suddenly, out of nowhere, thanks to two rather strange individuals who turned up at her house and spoke with her husband, most probably in private, suddenly everything was up in the air again and she was told she had to up sticks overnight and move. I can imagine the heavy heart and dragging feet with which she set off. I'm sure she had a serious discussion with Lot about it all during that final night she slept in her home, but in the end, those two strangers literally dragged them out of the house and on to the road out of the city. As she walked away, she must have thought about all that she had built up in Sodom and all that she had left behind, and she did what anyone would do. She took a last lingering look back at what she had left.

Lot's wife turned to a pillar of salt because she didn't accept what she had been told about the fate of the city she had come to call home and what she needed to do to escape it. Lot believed what he had been told by those strangers and so should she, but she found it too difficult. She wasn't prepared to look forward to a future with her husband and family without looking back at a life she didn't want to leave behind. Despite the seedy, debauched underbelly of a city that she knew Sodom was, it was home. Looking back at it cost her her life, Lot his wife and their daughters their mother. It resulted in Lot's wife's lasting legacy being a warning to humanity of what not to do.

We should not be individuals who are so focused on looking back on a life we are not prepared to give up that we can't see the life God has destined us to live with Him in the future.

I had an image of a cold, porous statue of myself looking back over the hills and valleys that had been my life and of the rains of my current situation dripping on it until it ran away in foul, briny channels. While the vastness of my future lay before me, because I was turned the wrong way, I couldn't see it and, if truth be told, I didn't want to. I was living a lesser life, and by implication was forcing Ralph to live a lesser life with me. Rather than looking forward to what God was going to bring both of us in this 'D' life of now, I was looking back with unrealistic fondness at a life I thought was preferable to the one I was currently living.

When I was a teenager and going to coffee bars which were the Christian gathering places of my youth, very often speakers would tell us that God was not finished with us (Philippians 1:6); that He had much more in store for us if we would just trust Him. I believe that is true of every generation and age, not just of youth, and true for every individual regardless of their ability or disabilities. I had lived a full and meaningful life up until the 'D' diagnosis, but it wasn't over. I was taking Ralph's diagnosis on myself and assuming that it meant the end of my life as I understood my life to be. But that wasn't what God wanted. There was more life to come with every breath and minute and day that God in His divine providence would give me. If I kept looking back, how could I ever see what He had in store for me in the future?

I also realised, however, that God was not done with Ralph. Just because Ralph had this 'D' diagnosis and now was starting on this 'D' part of his life journey, it didn't mean that God was finished with him. He had more life to experience, more blessings to receive and give, and while he might at times – and increasingly in the future – live in his past life, that didn't mean he couldn't enjoy his life now and have meaningful and happy days, weeks and, in God's will, years in the future.

I resolved not to wilfully look back any more. I was so grateful for the life that I had lived, so thankful for the blessings of work and achievement, so in awe of the wonderful husband God had given me when I least expected it, but also so aware that there was so much more to come. The boundary lines of my life up until this point really had been drawn for me in 'pleasant places', but those 'pleasant places' hadn't and wouldn't end with Ralph's dementia diagnosis. There was more life to come, and I needed to look forward so that I could see it and experience all that God wanted me and Ralph to enjoy in it.

Looking back on that list of the ten worst things that had ever happened in my life, I knew that if I were to write a new list now, Ralph's 'D' diagnosis would rank very high up and, if I were honest, over the coming years it was likely to go up that list as I rewrote it, not down. While I had to accept that now, and in the months and years ahead of us in God's will, it was always going to be the giant that stalked both of us, I resolved that I was going to do my utmost to keep it where it needed to be. I would keep this giant of dementia in front of me and Ralph and, with God's help and grace, we would face it together.

There could not and would not be any more looking back at my previous life. God had not finished with me and God had not finished with Ralph. There was so much more to come for both of us, of that I was absolutely certain, and I wasn't going to miss a minute of it, for either of us.

3
Learning to Share

When I was in my late twenties, in the mid-1980s, I worked for three years in Nepal with an international mission organisation. For two of those years I lived and worked with a fellow Ulsterwoman in a small village in the Gorkha region in the middle hills of Nepal, three hours from the mission's hospital that served as our base. The hospital in turn was three hours' trek from a main road where we could catch a bus into Kathmandu and the mission headquarters.

After I had been there for some months, I began to get used to trekking everywhere, as the village we lived in was situated at more than 5,000ft above sea level and we worked in surrounding villages up to 8,000ft. One weekend, we both headed back to the mission hospital for a weekend with friends there. To my extreme shock, I discovered after arriving at the hospital that I had left something important in our village home that I really needed and that there was nothing else for it but to go back to the village to get it the following day. I knew that meant I had to walk there and back in one day, something I had never done before. Despite the inconvenience, I was content to do this as I was extremely fit from all the walking on the hills and rice terraces that had become part and parcel of my everyday village life. So, early the next morning, I set off by myself to walk back to the village, not thinking it necessary to take a porter or guide for company or safety. This was long before the advent of mobile phones and instant communication.

A memorable companion

As I began my walk, I actually enjoyed the stillness of a misty morning which was so typical of days in the middle hills of Nepal at that time of the year. Walking by myself, with no significant backpack, carrying only water and some snacks for the journey, I made it back to the village in record time. I retrieved the item that I needed, took a rest in our little home over midday, and when the sun had started its descent, set off to walk back to the mission hospital, with every expectation that I would make it well before sunset.

Less than one hour into my return journey I began to experience pain in both ankles, and by the time I had reached the midway point of the trek, I was in real agony. Each step was causing jolting pains in my ankles that were spreading up my legs and into my hips. It became so bad that I was almost crying with pain every step I took. I eventually made it to a small village which signified what we called the last stage of the journey to the hospital. From this point, under normal circumstances, it was a thirty-minute steady uphill climb on a well-formed mud path interspersed with slabs of rock that had been dug into the hill. These formed much-appreciated steps for travellers climbing them, who were often carrying children or adults to the hospital to get the medical treatment they needed.

I literally collapsed under a large tree at the centre of the village, where many a weary traveller took rest, and sat there hugging my aching legs, rubbing my ankles and wondering how on earth I was going to make it up the hill. I could see that the sun was going down rapidly. It was now late afternoon and I knew that if I didn't get up the hill in the next hour, I wouldn't make it back to the hospital before sunset. I was debating with myself whether I should try to pay a villager to go up to the hospital with a message for someone to come down and get me and carry me up like a patient. Or should I try to find a room in a house in the village where the owners would let me stay overnight and, hopefully, I would be fit to do the walk in the morning? While the people I had met on the path up to this point were sympathetic as they realised I was in great pain, there was understandable reticence on their part about helping a single woman, especially a foreign one, so I knew it was not going to be easy to get help.

As I was trying to work out what to do, I became aware of a shadow at the corner of my vision, and when I looked up, standing about twenty yards to my right was a small Nepali woman. She was just an ordinary village woman, barefooted and in typical Gorkhali dress, but, unusually, she was by herself, with no children or other women with her. She was standing between me and the beginning of the path up to the hospital, but she was looking directly at me. As I focused on her, I had the most amazing sense of peace and calmness and I could not help but keep my gaze on her for a number of seconds. Then suddenly she broke eye contact with me, turned around and headed up the path.

As I watched, she stopped, turned, again looked directly at me and said, 'Come.' She said it in the lowest form of the Nepali language verb. The form you would use to say 'come' to a pet or a small child. She said it a couple of times and gestured with her hand for me to come towards her. I shook my head and all but cried when saying to her, in Nepali, that I couldn't come, that my legs were too sore. She turned, walked another few steps, turned and again said, 'Come,' and waited.

It seemed like several minutes passed but it was only several seconds until again she said, 'Come,' and waited. I got up and literally hobbled towards her, thinking that she must be offering to help me up the hill, but just as I got to within touching distance of her, she turned around and set off. I couldn't believe it. I had walked towards her for help and she had turned her back on me and walked away. I stopped where I was and just looked at her back, nearly falling down with the pain. Just as I was going to hobble back to the tree, she walked towards me, got within touching distance again, stared directly into my eyes and said, 'Come, little one, come.' I hobbled off towards her and once again, just when I got near her, she turned and headed off up the hill.

This scenario repeated itself for more than one hour as she walked in front of me the entire way up the hill. Waiting for me when the pain got too much and I had to rest, and then even though I would have waited longer, she always said, 'Come, little one,' and we set off again. When we eventually got to the top of the hill just as the sun was going down, she waited for me to get right up close to her, smiled, gave a shake of her head as a parting gesture and turned and walked briskly away, not looking back. I was in such pain I could hardly speak, but called after her, 'Thank you, big sister.' That journey and that woman have stayed in my memory for decades, and always will.

Personal time for me

My new-found intention to look forward to all that God had in store for me coincided with a planned meeting with our social worker in June 2017. I had presumed it would be the usual type of meeting with her and expected to have conversations about Ralph's disease progression and future service needs as his health and mental state deteriorated. However, to my great surprise, the meeting was all about me. We discussed how I was feeling about the current and future situation with his health, and what plans I had in place to ensure that my own physical and mental health remained strong and resilient. She felt that since things with Ralph had now settled down into more of a pattern, it was important that I formulated plans for me as an individual, and in particular thought about trying to set aside some personal time each week. She asked about my friends and family and what support I got from them. She was keen to learn what interests I had and how I pursued them.

Owing to my career path in early life, I had spent a number of years outside Northern Ireland, first at college in Scotland and then five years working abroad. College and school friends had long since gone and the reality was that Ralph was my best and only real friend. During the twenty-six years of our marriage up to the point of Ralph's diagnosis, we had been entirely self-sufficient in each other, with only very few other people in our lives, apart from his children who were all grown up with families of their own. It was a situation we had enjoyed, if not actively encouraged, particularly over the previous two years when it had been very evident to me that Ralph was developing memory loss and some unusual social habits and actions, which did not bode well when we were with other people.

We had in some regards retreated into a very self-contained life, totally centred on each other, so it was a very strange situation to be thinking about a life for me that didn't primarily focus on Ralph. The social worker suggested that I should start to have some 'me' time each week and advised that I could get a sitter to come for a few hours to allow me to go out of the house by myself, meet up with friends or do something specifically for me, while they stayed in the home and kept a watchful eye on Ralph.

At first, I was very against this. I couldn't think of what on earth I would want to do without Ralph, let alone where I would go to do it. However, something she said to me really struck home. She said that if Ralph's physical health continued to deteriorate as it had been doing rapidly in recent months, it would come to a point where I physically would not be able to care for him by myself.

I was going to need at the very least some help, and at the very most my care for him would require total replacement by trained carers coming into the home, perhaps a number of times each day. I had to agree with her that such a situation would be very invasive in our home and lives. As we talked, she gently helped me to see that it could be less intrusive to start off with some small service to get us both used to others being involved in Ralph's care. We also talked about the role of his family in his care and that while it was admirable that I wanted to do everything for him, I was actually excluding them from being involved. This meant that I was reducing their input into their father's life at a stage when he still for the most part was able to recognise and feel comfortable with them and their own families.

I left that meeting with the realisation that perhaps once again I had been somewhat selfish in my attitude, wanting if not needing to do everything for Ralph myself to prove that I could. But also, if I was honest, I did it to keep others out. I had no other job or purpose right then but to be with and care for Ralph, and so I did all of it myself, as to do otherwise might be to admit that my life was devoid of any other real meaning. Shades of my previous insecurities about my last job obviously were still with me.

As I thought about all that the social worker had said, I knew that she was right. I needed to let others in, both family and others, to share in Ralph's care, but also to share in my care and my life. I needed to keep looking forward, of course, but I also needed to look to see who else was in the wings, waiting and wanting to provide both Ralph and me with support and encouragement as we travelled along this 'D' journey. This wouldn't negate what I was doing, but rather would be a validation that I was doing things well and was on the right path. However, I needed to accept that there were others who could walk with me on this path and help share the load. They would not take over, but rather, by their presence and appropriate actions, would provide support to both Ralph and me. They could walk behind me, waiting to catch me if I fell. They could walk ahead of me to prepare the path I would need to travel, and they could lead me to the next stop on my care journey. Most of all, they could walk beside me to let me know that I was not alone but that this was a shared journey which they were willing and wanting to be a part of.

Accepting support from others

Over the years of our marriage, I had grown especially close to Ralph's three daughters, Lynda, Gwen and Wilma. They became and are friends and confidantes. When Ralph's physical health began to deteriorate, really from as far back as 2005 when his mobility was seriously reduced owing to osteoarthritis in his spine, they were only too well aware of his advancing years and had been supporting us both as his health progressively worsened. Even after I had retired, in the years before his diagnosis they had frequently come to stay with him for a few hours while I went out to do some shopping, and after his diagnosis this became a regular occurrence. I appreciated their help and support so much and was content to accept this from family, but it seemed a big leap to have to now accept help from outside the family. However, they and his two sons were fully supportive of me taking advantage of this service. All his children told me again and again that if I wanted to continue to support their dad and keep him at home with me, I needed to keep myself healthy, not just physically but also mentally, and having even a couple of hours to myself every week would help me in this.

So I accepted the sitter service, and a couple of weeks later someone arrived on a specified afternoon to stay with Ralph while I went out. The first couple of weeks I was like a lost soul wandering around. I genuinely did not know what to do with myself. The first week that the service was in place, I stayed with the sitter for the first hour and then, when Ralph seemed content enough, I went out to do a bit of shopping for the two hours of agreed time left.

Thirty minutes later the needed shopping was done. I had walked in and out of a few shops that I might not normally have gone into to look at things I didn't need. I realised that because over the previous few years I had never had the time to browse in shops, always being aware that Ralph was sitting in the car waiting for me to return, I had forgotten how to look and linger as part of the shopping process. I also discovered that I felt unusually self-conscious walking around by myself with no actual shopping to do.

I bought myself an ice cream and went back to the car to eat it in glorious solitude. As I licked my ice cream and listened to the radio, I reflected on the choices I was making at this time in our shared dementia journey. I realised that I had declined help and support to the point where I had wilfully excluded others who would have willingly helped me, and in doing so had isolated Ralph and me from them. Our lives were lesser because of my desire to do everything, lonelier because of my insistence that we were enough in ourselves and smaller because of our – or, more truthfully, my – limited vision. I was still hankering after past ways or, at the very most, looking only a very few steps ahead in our journey. I needed not just to look up and see what was ahead, but also to look sideways to see who else was waiting in the wings of our lives and accept help from them in whatever form it came – to allow others to help us both along this 'D' journey we were travelling on.

Over the weeks that followed, I came to look forward to my afternoons off, as I described them. Everyone in the family was particularly pleased to see that this sitter service was in place because they recognised that it gave me some time to myself to recharge my resilience batteries and put my life in perspective. When they could, Lynda, Gwen and Wilma met up with me on those afternoons and took me out to shop or to have coffee or lunch. But having the sitter service in place didn't mean the girls stopped coming to give me other times to have a break.

Wilma came and sat with her dad on an occasional Sunday night while I went to church. That was a wonderful gift and I so appreciated it, but it was also a special time for her to be with her father. Lynda and I met up for a walk in a local park every few weeks, which usually ended with a coffee or an ice cream. Gwen often turned up at the house at the weekend with a lovely bunch of flowers to brighten our home, and I could go out for a time knowing that Ralph was safe. They all phoned regularly, came to visit, spent time with their dad and always encouraged me to go out and do some shopping or take a walk as an extra time gift when they were with him.

However, these times also provided opportunities for me to talk with each of them, about their dad, of course, but also about their lives and my life and the things that were important to us all. Through those precious times I grew closer to them in ways I might otherwise not have done, as often when they came to our home their purpose and their conversation was understandably all about Ralph. I got to know them all better as women and as friends, and over the weeks and months following his diagnosis our relationships grew and deepened in a way that I never expected but so valued.

These afternoons off were also the means by which I began to regain some of the self-confidence and self-belief that I had lost over the previous two years since my retirement from full-time employment. I had been such a strong woman throughout my career, with a broad spectrum of work-related interests and commitments. To go from that life to one that had become so insular and constrained by the nature of Ralph's deteriorating condition had sapped my confidence in a way that I had not fully appreciated. I had become a woman who walked with her head down, not up, who spoke rarely when I was out of the house, who never lingered or browsed but who did what needed to be done in as short a time as possible and then retreated back into the safety of her home.

This 'me' time also provided much-needed stimulus and variation in our shared lives. When I came back home, I chatted to Ralph about things I had done on my afternoons away, the people I had seen, the things I had bought, where I had had a coffee. I told him about the conversations I had with the girls, even if at times he had to be reminded who they were. He sometimes even laughed and smiled when I shared anecdotes and experiences of them and their children that they had shared with me. The increasing confidence I gained over this time enabled me to share him with his family and others and to share me with them. In doing so, I believe that both Ralph and I learned to walk along and cope better with the 'D' life and the journey we were now on together. As a consequence of this gift of time for me and the people who gave it to me, I became a better person and a better carer.

I liked me better.

4
Our Journey Gets More Difficult

The Giraffe
There was a giraffe on the high street today
Standing in a parking spot outside the bank.
It looked down on you, you said
With its big dark eyes and winked.
You laughed as you told me.
I saw a motorcycle.

What pretty tulips you said
As I put the roses on the table.
With their tall stems and waxy petals, they're
    almost regal
The Queen will like them when she comes to
    tea today.
As the doorbell rang you tried to get up in
    deference to her
As the sitter walked in.

I envy you your wonderment
To be able to see the extraordinary in the
    mundane.

Magic in the routine that has become your life
Your mind, shrinking and dying, still hopes,
    and dreams.
Did you see it, you said, wasn't it amazing?
Of course I saw it. How could you miss a
    giraffe?

Five months post-diagnosis and the 'D' journey was getting harder for both of us. It started with Ralph just staring at me silently for a few minutes without blinking. Then his speech would become slower until it would get to the point where he would be unable to get any words out, which totally frustrated him to the point that he became very agitated. This was followed by him becoming completely withdrawn from me and others. These changes quickly degenerated into what I came to call his 'zoned-out' state.

Zoning-out times

This zoned-out state was usually preceded by Ralph sleeping even more than what I had come to understand was normal for him. He was spending more and more of each day sleeping or dozing. He went quiet. He stopped talking to me. He wouldn't answer questions and he just stared. His blank eyes were so deep and unflinching, staring past me, not at me. Ralph's focus seemed to be beyond me to a place on the wall or outside the window, and often I thought he was staring at a place where I was not. I even wondered if he knew who I was at these times. But after a few seconds or several minutes he would blink, look at me and then say that of course he knew me. For those few seconds I had glimpses of what our future would be like.

And then Ralph fell. Inevitable, really, but shocking nevertheless. In actual fact, it was not so much a fall as a glide. As I told his children later, he slid gracefully to the floor like a dying swan. Quieter, too. Unfortunately, it happened when I was showering him and I had to call for help to get him up once I was satisfied that he had not broken anything, a fact that was later confirmed by a home visit from our doctor. I think what annoyed Ralph most was that his son-in-law saw him with no clothes on, typically embarrassed and shy man that he is! That fall showed me that not only was Ralph's mind deteriorating, his physical state was also. I noticed how small he was becoming and how much I could feel his bones through his clothes. When I hugged him and snuggled my head into his chest, I could not help but see that my head was now at the same level as his and, despite my best efforts, he had lost quite a bit of weight, which meant that I no longer had to bend over his tummy to rest my head against him.

At first these zoned-out phases only came and went every few weeks, but as time passed they became more frequent and then increasingly severe. Ralph stared for hours. He didn't close his eyes when he lay down to rest, and he would lie for hours on the bed staring into space. During these times he blinked rarely and did not respond to conversation. When pressed, he would respond to repeated questions, if somewhat reluctantly and with poor grace, as if I had interrupted him and disturbed his train of thought. I couldn't content myself being away from him when he was experiencing one of these episodes. I even started to stock up on some essentials just in case I couldn't get to the shops. My freezer became full of meals and bread and vegetables and potato products. I knew I could always nip to the filling station shop just up the road if I was desperate for milk, but I wasn't going to be caught short running out of food.

When Ralph came out of these zoned-out episodes, he could say meaningful words and knew he had experienced, as he described it, a bad time or a bad day, but he couldn't explain how he had felt during that time. He just knew it hadn't been good and he didn't like it. When I pressed him on how he had felt during the bad time, he just used words like 'awful' and 'terrible' and talked about his head not being right. When he did return to me, as I described it, he was bright and responsive and actually had more energy. He was keen to get out in the car, to go for coffee and could engage in meaningful conversation about our life or his children's lives. But then it would come back and he would be away in his own world again, isolated and alone. I worried that one day he would never come back to me from this solitary world he now found himself in more often.

The other surprising trait Ralph developed at this stage was a fascination with his hands, fingers and arms. I would wake up in the night to find him lying on his back, head up, with one or sometimes two arms outstretched and moving one or both hands almost as if he were conducting an orchestra. While he did this, his lips were moving but no sound was coming out, and most surprising of all to me was the fact that he was also elegantly moving his fingers, almost in time to music that he was hearing in his mind. At other times while he was sleeping, I would see him lifting his arm up and pointing his finger and then he would smile or laugh to himself, as he was obviously seeing something that made him happy.

When he was awake, he liked to hold my hand and would gently stroke it or rub my palm with his thumb and look into my eyes and smile. The senses of touching and feeling became so important to Ralph at this time. He got really upset when the tap water was too hot or too cold for him. He noticed the coarseness of his trousers compared to the softness of his jumper, and he hated a rough towel. I ended up putting his bath towel in the tumble dryer before I showered him so that it was warm and soft for him. He would hold it around himself for a few seconds and smile at the pleasure he felt from this simple gesture.

All the children and grandchildren noticed this decline and did not like it. They came to accept that sometimes when they came to see him, he just did not know who they were in relation to him. On one occasion, when his eldest daughter, Lynda, had left after spending a couple of hours with him, he asked me who the nice lady was who had come to see him. When I told him it was his daughter, he laughed and said he didn't have any daughters. I would take time to go over and over the names of his children and grandchildren, but sadly he could not always remember them and often questioned who they all were. The times when he knew them, interacted with them and held their hands or hugged them became very precious, something both they and I treasured.

It was at this stage in our 'D' journey that Ralph even began to have problems knowing where he was at times. Sometimes he would head off to the wrong room in our home. I lost him a few times and found him sitting in a spare bedroom, and when I asked him where he was, he admitted he didn't know but thought this was a nice room and asked me if he could stay there. Sometimes he would wake up out of a nap or sleep and say he wanted to go home. When I asked him where he thought he was, he would say he didn't know. When I asked him where home was, he would just look at me and say nothing. I told him he was home, that this was his home, our home, but he genuinely looked puzzled and unbelieving. He came with me for a walk around it but I could see the incredulity in his eyes that he was here and not where he thought he should be.

Sometimes when I went to get Ralph up for a meal, he would say he didn't want to go down to the dining room, or that he wasn't dressed for dinner. I realised that he thought he was in a hotel. Quite a compliment, I used to think, that our home was up to hotel standards, but frightening that he didn't recognise where he was and wanted to go to another place, a safer place, a more familiar place. He started to ask me frequently who was in the house, why there was only the two of us for dinner and where everyone else was. Wherever he was, here with me was not home, not familiar and not identifiable as part of his history, let alone his present. It saddened me to think that he wanted to be somewhere else or that he wanted to be with other people, or to have them with him. I worried he was unhappy, discontent or ill at ease with me and with us.

I thought of how much time was now being spent in these zoned-out states and, as a consequence, how much less real time we had together. I began to dread these zoned-out times. They came almost weekly and so, for up to one day each week, Ralph would be away in a far-off place, far from me and far from others. It seemed that no matter how hard I tried, I couldn't reach him. He was beyond me and also, I felt, beyond himself. I only hoped that wherever he was, he was not unhappy or distressed and that when he returned, he could find some rest and peace.

Throughout our married life we had spent every minute we could together, content in and with each other. We enjoyed family get-togethers for birthdays, special events and summer barbecues and we enjoyed fellowship in the church we attended, but we were like two halves of the one whole and very content in that. These zoned-out times made me realise that our close union was beginning to separate. Ralph was slowly being drawn away from me by this awful disease and there was absolutely nothing I could do about it.

The times the locusts ate

I begrudged these times. They were wasted times, waiting times, in my mind. It was as if our lives were on hold until Ralph came out of them. I thought of the passage in the book of Joel where it talks about the 'years the locusts have eaten' (Joel 2:25) and it seemed to really describe what I felt was happening to us both:

> What the locust swarm has left
> the great locusts have eaten;
> what the great locusts have left
> the young locusts have eaten;
> what the young locusts have left
> other locusts have eaten.
> *Joel 1:4*

The wretched locust of dementia was eating away at the life we had, and no matter how hard we tried to stop it, it just carried on. When I took the time to look up the reference in a more contemporary paraphrase of the Bible, it described a range of locusts that just came along one after another to eat what the previous ones had left behind until there was absolutely nothing left at all. They chewed, gobbled and munched their way through all the grain fields that were in front of them until there was nothing left, only bare and barren land:

> What the chewing locust left,
> the gobbling locust ate;
> What the gobbling locust left,
> the munching locust ate;
> What the munching locust left,
> the chomping locust ate.
> *Joel 1:4 (The Message)*

Not a pleasant comparison with our current situation, if truth be told, but probably an appropriate description of where Ralph was at this stage, his brain somewhere between chewed and munched and heading towards all gobbled up. The inexorable decline of his cognitive and memory functions was well on its way, and I had the awful feeling that more locusts were waiting in the wings to see it through to the end. I could only hope and pray that one day, somehow, we would have this time back and that Ralph would have his mind back.

I started my scribblings again, and this time I didn't delete them, but rather doubled up on them. When some event or comment Ralph made, or an experience that we had together moved me, I wrote it down and then I sat back and thought about what I had written. Where had it come from? Where did I want it to take my thoughts to, my life to, and his life to? And when I had rationalised it in my mind, I wrote a second complementary scribble reflecting that journey. I gave them titles. Rather presumptive, I know, but it was done to define a time, a situation and a halting point in the journey; to mark it for me, in the realisation that one day I would look back and read it and remember that time.

'The Giraffe' poem above and 'A Free Fight' poem below reflect that scribbling journey, and are markers of an event and of a time which I will always have of Ralph. Their titles are anagrams of each other and that in itself is a consequence of my thinking at this time. Did he see the giraffe? Ralph believed he did and I believe him. I didn't see it, but then perhaps I was so intent on doing my shopping in the town as quickly as possible that I missed it. Was it a real giraffe? I can't believe it was as there were no reports of stray giraffes roaming around our local town that day, but perhaps while Ralph was waiting for me to return from the bank, he saw a child walking by the car carrying a cuddly toy giraffe. Or perhaps he saw a children's play bus go by which had animals painted on the side. However Ralph saw it, he saw a giraffe and it made him smile and he remembered it long enough to tell me about it when I returned to the car, and that made *me* smile.

As I reflected on this later, I thought about all the processes in his mind that must have made him see that giraffe and think that it interacted with him, and so I wrote the second complementary piece below to try to rationalise these processes to myself and help me contextualise them in the overall state of his 'D' life. Ralph was changing in front of me from the man I knew and loved, and at this time in our 'D' journey I was struggling to both understand the changes and accept them. I knew God would never 'ordain' them, but they were happening, and this poem reflects my inner turmoil at witnessing them.

However, the progression in Ralph's condition and the decline we were all seeing was only our view of him and his condition on this 'D' journey. While we saw him deteriorate and his memory and cognitive ability fail as evidenced by less verbal and social interaction with us, Ralph increasingly saw and engaged in an entirely different world. A new world. A world of music and laughter. A world he was actively involved in, even conducting, pointing out significant events, milestones and markers to himself and others. Ralph could see giraffes and nice ladies. He stayed in hotels and had no commitments. He saw people he recognised and places he wanted to be, and he experienced times he could laugh at and enjoy.

In the main, he was content and happy in these places and did not need others with him. He was sometimes even able to share these experiences with me. Such times made me realise that there were two views, two experiences of this 'D' journey. One wasn't better than the other, or of any less importance. Both were real and valid experiences, and probably the sum of them together gave a better reflection of this journey that we were all on than we would admit. We were all – Ralph, me and his family – active travellers on this road. Walking as individuals, of course, but also walking with each other and sharing some experiences along the way, but not all. The reality of it was that I and the family needed to come to a place where we accepted that we couldn't or, indeed, didn't need to share each and every experience that Ralph had on his 'D' journey. Where some of us saw giraffes, others saw motorcycles. Where some saw decline and fragility, others saw our history and where we had come from. Where some of us had a better insight into where we might be going, others were not concerned about this at all and were just totally focused on enjoying the part of the journey we were now on.

There were, of course, parts of Ralph's journey that he was not able to actively engage in. The zoned-out times when he couldn't interact with or share with others or me and the solitary or fearful times. All I could hope was that he would know that he was not alone at these times; that I, his family and others were with him and that we would wait for him to come back to us so that we could all walk on together. Most of all, I prayed that Ralph would know that God was with him at these times, that he would sense His presence with him, even in those most lonely and frightening of zoned-out times.

Our shared 'D' journey would, of course, have its ups and downs, its level, smooth sections and its rocky hill climbs, but we were all on the same road and would eventually arrive at the same destination. We all just needed to accept that, like any journey, each of us on it would see different things and have different experiences on the way that we could share and relive both at the current time and in the future. Even if Ralph could not always share his memories with me, I wanted and needed to have memories of this time. Such shared experiences are what lasting memories are made of, and one thing I knew for certain, I definitely wanted and needed to have a full barn of shared memories of the good times and even the not-so-good times we had and were having. I needed to store them up and keep them safe so that I would have them to draw on and relish in the future.

A Free Fight
Was it ordained from before time began
That life's path would wind this way for you?
A crack appeared and stopped a leap, a jump
And became more cracks upon cracks that
    crisscrossed
To become a lake, a flatland, a mesh
Through which nothing jumped or leapt but
    sank.

People became colours and food had sounds.
Family became foe and strangers, friends.

Fear masked as laughter and embarrassment
    relinquished.
Now became then, sooner was later and never
    was unknown.
No one in the driving seat of your life
Free falling with no resistance.

What were the odds, who cast the lots and
    threw the dice
That tumbled and jumbled and slipped and
    felled you
Into a life without boundaries or fetters or
    chains?
Redefining happiness, redrawing lines.
Impossible to fight, or change or sigh.
Was it lost before it began?

5

The Road Narrows

When we were first married, in the early 1990s, Ralph and I really enjoyed spending time together without always needing the company of friends or family. Somewhat selfish, perhaps, but nevertheless happiness and contentment for us.

These were the days before online booking sites and hotel comparison sites, and we would often scour the newspaper on a Friday night for any offers that local hotels might advertise for weekend or midweek breaks. Sometimes you could get one or two nights' bed and breakfast with an evening meal at a reasonable price in a good, if not *very* good, hotel, and we would take advantage of these offers every couple of months. As time progressed, we managed to buy and sell a number of properties up on the north coast of Northern Ireland, and enjoyed using those for holidays and weekend breaks. They provided a bolthole, an escape and a refuge from the pressures of life, work and challenging health issues for both Ralph and me. They were such good times. Walking together along beaches and harbour walls, sharing quality time with each other as we enjoyed beautiful scenery and even occasionally joining with friends who either also had properties up there or who came to stay with us.

Ralph had never really had what he would term 'foreign' holidays before he met me. While he had been to a couple of European countries in connection with his business, he never went on package holidays, organised walking holidays or city breaks. Even for our honeymoon I couldn't persuade him to book a holiday in Italy or Switzerland, which I would have loved to have seen. Instead we ended up in the Channel Islands because, as he commented, they spoke English and used pound notes. For my fortieth birthday, after much persuasion, Ralph reluctantly agreed to take me on a package holiday to Lanzarote and, to his complete amazement, he really enjoyed it. I had done the booking and had gone for the quieter option of a smaller town, smaller apartment block and no inclusive food, and it worked very well for a virgin package-holiday man.

As the years passed, though, Ralph began to have real problems walking, and gradually his mobility deteriorated to the point where he couldn't walk for any great distance and was uncomfortable sitting for any period of time. Plane journeys of anything more than an hour became impossible, and even negotiating the airports, with their interminable walking distances to departure gates, was just out of the question. We had enjoyed a number of holidays in warm climes over the first years of our marriage, but gradually they petered out as Ralph was unwilling to use a wheelchair to get from the car park to the airport terminal or from the check-in desk to the gate. I realised that it was pointless putting him through the pain of travelling just for the sake of a week or two in the sun, as it took him a few days to recover from the journey at both ends of the holiday.

So, as we moved into another decade of marriage, we rediscovered breaks and holidays at home. From our previous forays on the island, we had a number of hotels in both Northern Ireland and the Republic of Ireland that we really liked, so we holidayed there. We enjoyed good rooms, great food and enjoyable trips to local beauty spots; we shopped in new towns and rested and recouped from the pressures of life. Good times.

After I retired and a full year before Ralph's diagnosis, we managed to have two midweek breaks in a lovely hotel we had stayed in a number of times before. It was during the last time we stayed there that I really began to appreciate just how serious Ralph's mental decline had become. On our second day, we had booked an afternoon tea which was served in a very elegant conservatory. We presented ourselves at the desk to check in for our afternoon delight, and the waiter greeted us both and asked us to follow him to the table reserved for us. I was in front, so I set off following the waiter. A few moments later I reached our assigned table and began to set down my handbag and take off my jacket.

At this point the waiter inclined his head towards me and quietly asked, 'Is your husband not joining you?' I looked back at the reception desk and Ralph was standing there by himself looking totally lost. I excused myself and walked quickly back to the desk and asked him what was wrong and why he hadn't followed me.

He simply said, 'You didn't tell me to; you just left me here.'

I had never seen him look so alone, so afraid and so sad. I took his hand, walked him to our table and said how sorry I was that I had left him. We did take our afternoon tea together, but it was ruined for me as I saw how dependent, how vulnerable and how lost he had become.

A life without surprises

As time had progressed over the years of our marriage prior to my retirement, I had gradually taken over more and more of the organisation of our lives. I had continued to work full-time but took charge of paying the bills, saw to the maintenance and upkeep of the house, dealt with boiler men, electricians and painters and generally ran the home. Ralph, in contrast, had entered into a phase of his life where he waited. Waited for me to come home from work. Waited for the weekend when we could spend more time together and waited for others to come to him, to phone him, to talk to him and to engage with him. Meanwhile, I continued to work full-time, to keep the house and home and him and us, until eventually there was no other option but to take the very difficult decision to retire early, in 2015, and care for him full-time. Looking back, I now see that these years prior to his diagnosis were in essence a preparatory 'D' life phase.

Our history determines our present, which in turn determines our future. With hindsight I can now see so very clearly that the general deterioration in Ralph's health over the years prior to his dementia diagnosis, coupled with the change of responsibility for the organisation of our lives from him to me, was really the precursor and apprenticeship for the life we would both be forced to lead following his diagnosis. As I moved further into this new chosen role of a carer, I realised and accepted that my life to that point had been in no small part a preparation for this caring time.

What struck me very quickly about my new role as a full-time carer was that my life was now totally without surprise and surprises. There was no one to say on a Friday night, 'Don't bother cooking; let's go out for tea.' No one to say, 'Guess what, I've booked us a weekend away next month.' Never again would I find a gift on my bed for a birthday, or just for me. I organised everything, planned our lives and facilitated our living. Even before Ralph had received his final diagnosis, I had realised how bad things were becoming when I had to ask his daughter Wilma to take him out for an hour to buy me a Christmas card and gift because he couldn't do that himself. What was so sad was to know how much he would have hated that. Ralph was such a generous man, always spending far too much on me for birthdays and Christmas, and to have come to the stage where he couldn't even manage to do that himself would have been so hard for him to accept. When he did go out with her to get gifts, I had to give Wilma his wallet and she made the payments and transactions. For a businessman, this was the ultimate humiliation, not even being able to pay for a card for his wife. The only redeeming fact was that he very quickly got to the stage where he didn't even know that he was incapable of doing this simple task of love. Ralph just thought that she was buying the gifts and he was not entirely sure or didn't have a clue who they were for.

It was in September 2017, about six months after Ralph's diagnosis, that I suddenly saw how small and insular our lives now were. It now took hours to get both of us up and organised. I couldn't take any appointments or plan to do anything before ten o'clock in the morning because it was that time of the day before I could get us both up and dressed. By the time I had got Ralph up, given him his medication, got him shaved, showered or hair washed and then dressed and got him his breakfast, it was mid-morning at the earliest. I then just threw on whatever clothes were appropriate for the day and dragged a brush through my hair. By that stage I was exhausted. We continued to have certain regular events like coffee out on the same day every week by ourselves or with family, and he still sat in the car while I went into our local town or village to get groceries or do shopping, but in reality, our lives centred around our home and within a five-mile radius. It was becoming a real effort to get us out and about and the effort for both of us to do so sometimes seemed too much. This time coincided with Ralph having more frequent episodes of losing control of his bladder and I was panicky about him having an accident when we were in a coffee shop or in one of his children's homes.

Our spiritual journey narrows

It was also at this time that I had to accept how insular and narrow our spiritual lives were. From our wedding night on, Ralph and I had always read God's Word and prayed together every night. I always did the reading, using my preferred version of the Bible, the New International Version, and very often when I was reading the passage for the night in this version, Ralph would be quietly repeating it with me in his preferred version, which was, of course, given his generation, the Authorised (King James) Version. Ralph had been, I shall graciously say, encouraged to learn long portions of the Bible by rote as a child when he attended a Brethren Sunday school in the 1940s, and they were so well drilled into him that he could still quote them decades later. Our nightly Bible reading was often like a mismatched, discordant duet, 'thee' and 'thine' competing with 'you' and 'yours', 'only begotten' vying with 'one and only'[4] and 'finisher' with 'perfecter'.[5]

We had also always prayed together nightly, originally taking it in turns. Ralph was a great man of prayer, and by that I mean a man of great long prayers! As well as praying for us and our situations, he had a very long list of individuals and topics he prayed for. He prayed nightly for each of his children and grandchildren by name. Ralph often used what I considered wonderfully old-fashioned terminology in his prayers. He prayed that his grandchildren would not 'make shipwreck of their lives', that they would 'walk the straight and narrow road' and of course that 'they would be saved'. Ralph always prayed at length for the church that we attended. In many churches, regardless of the denomination, it is common for people to sit in the same pew every week, and so he would start at the back of the church on one side and work his

---

[4] John 3:16 (NIV/AKJV).
[5] Hebrews 12:2 (NIV/AKJV).

way up and down, pew by pew, family by family, naming names where he could and describing individuals where he couldn't.

In addition to quoting Scripture at length, he had a vast repertoire of memorised verses from hymns and choruses and he would pepper his prayers with these in appropriate places. At times I marvelled at his memory of verse, Scripture and the people and situations he prayed for. I must admit, though, that at other times I wished he would speed up a bit, especially when I was working and just wanted to get to sleep to rest before the challenges of the next day. It was not unusual for Ralph to pray in excess of thirty minutes at night, and that was in addition to his personal prayers in the morning when I was at work, which I knew would be at least sixty to ninety minutes. On some nights when I prayed, I would take about five to ten minutes, and many times when I had finished, Ralph would gently take me by the hand and say that someone or some situation was on his heart and I had failed to mention them, so he would then pray for them for another ten minutes!

Over the years from Ralph's first signs of the reduction in his mobility, he had stopped going to church because he couldn't cope with the long service and having to sit on hard pews. Then, as his mental decline became more severe, he just couldn't concentrate and couldn't be still to listen. I had gone by myself for a number of months, but as time passed it was evident that he didn't want me to leave him, and so my own regular attendance dropped off significantly. We got tapes of the church services and listened to those for a while, watched services on the television and occasionally listened to the Sunday morning service on the radio, but very quickly Ralph stopped wanting to listen to them. He just couldn't follow a prayer or an illustration, never mind concentrate on a full sermon.

To my shame, I had, as the months went by following Ralph's diagnosis, become really lax about doing a nightly Scripture reading. By the time I got him prepared for and into bed and then myself sorted, he was fast asleep and it seemed pointless to read and pray out loud by myself. He seemed so far away from me, so unable to follow, at times, what I was saying, especially at night after he had taken his nightly medication, that I didn't see the point. I began to wonder how Ralph reached God and, indeed, if and how God reached him. Our shared spiritual lives were a thing of the past, and while I continued with my own personal quiet time, I missed our shared joint readings, his long prayers, his lines from choruses and the old-fashioned terminology of his memorised Bible verses.

I had to accept that our spiritual path had narrowed. Whereas before we had an active spiritual life in our church, now there were just the two of us on this quiet journey. I thought that was sad and sorrowful and restrictive. I missed collective worship as I didn't want to leave Ralph and only got to church occasionally when one of his daughters could come to stay with him. They would have done this more frequently than I asked, but I felt bad about asking them as it meant that they missed their own church services.

We did have visitors from our own church – we were so blessed by the couple who came, and who were so empathetic and encouraging to us both – but the solitary Christian life is almost a contradiction in itself and I missed fellowship, singing and Bible teaching. I could only try to imagine what must be going on in Ralph's mind, to have been unable to worship or to break bread and not to be with the fellowship of believers for so very long.

The lost sheep

As I thought about spiritually where we had both come from, had been and were now, I was reminded of the parable Jesus told about the shepherd looking for his lost sheep (Luke 15:1-7).

When I was a child, we had sheep for a short time on the farm I grew up on, and my father always thought of them as fickle animals. They would wander away and become lost or disorientated and he would have to go after them, across ditches or drains, and pull them out and get them back to the flock. What always worried me as a child was what would have happened if Dad hadn't gone to look for them. Would they have just continued to wander and get more and more disorientated to the point that they would have been totally lost and at the mercy of the elements or predators? I knew, however, that my father would never have allowed that to happen. Being the caring shepherd farmer that he was, he checked on his flocks and herds every day, and if there was an issue with a wandering or lost animal he would have immediately dropped everything else to go in search of it and return it to the safety that was the flock, the farm and himself.

God, as shepherd, comforted me at this time of spiritual lostness. I knew that God was out actively looking for us both as we were wandering, in my case, and being taken, in Ralph's case, away from our spiritual journey as we had known it in the past. I had a calm assurance and confidence that God had found Ralph where he was in his dementia and had been and was with him now, on his 'D' journey. I had a fresh awareness at this time that God was and is able to meet with individuals at the point of their need, in the state where they are, and in the abilities or disabilities that they have. As the world might assess the personal and corporate effectiveness of worship, fellowship and prayer, Ralph was completely unable to participate in or benefit from them. But he was with God, in God, and God was in him. Of that I was certain.

I dusted off the Authorised Bible. I dug out his *Believers Hymn Book* and I started to read to Ralph again nightly passages from God's Word in his familiar version. Even when he was sleeping, I read him verses from hymns that he would have sung as a child. I hoped that they would reach the recesses of his mind and bring him peace and comfort. It was an absolute joy when sometimes I would hear Ralph whisper a word in the passage, or move his lips along with my reading of a hymn. I prayed briefly after reading and sometimes he did manage an 'Amen', but even if he didn't, I was certain the words read and prayed brought him peace and comfort. What surprised me was how much comfort they brought me. Once again, we were joined together in our own worship, and simple and brief as it was, it was ours. Ralph's, mine and God's together.

The road didn't seem so narrow after all.

6
Time Passes By So Quickly

As autumn 2017 glided into winter, time slipped by. Hours became days, days became weeks which then relentlessly crept forward into months. It seemed to be but a breath from when I put Ralph's weekly medications in the little plastic pill boxes on a Saturday night until I was popping out his tablets into them again and realising that a full week had gone by.

There were good times and there were the inevitable bad times. There was a particularly bad week in late October when the combination of a urinary tract infection and a period of being zoned out just took him completely away from me. He didn't speak to me for three days. His eyes were scarily wide open and unblinking and he looked terrified as he obviously didn't recognise me or know where he was. He even slept with his eyes open, as if he was afraid to close them and submit to the darkness and lostness he must have been feeling. He was completely disorientated around the house, not knowing where to go and not recognising anything when he got there. He was uncoordinated, unable to feed himself because he couldn't work out how to get the food from his plate onto a fork and into his mouth. It was a fight to get him dressed as he tried to work out how to get arms into shirt sleeves and feet into slippers. I gave up after the first day and left him in his pyjamas and dressing gown. When he eventually emerged from this frightening state, he spoke virtual gibberish for a day and had unintelligible conversations with himself and me for the next few days. Eventually he steadied again and amazingly said to me, 'I'm not the man I was.' It broke my heart.

Once again after such a mind-bending event he then had a period of near lucidity for a few days when he was back to the husband and partner I knew. We resumed our drives out and about and enjoyed the ubiquitous coffee and scones. We even had rational conversations about how physically and mentally frail he had become, and dipped our toes into discussions about what would become of him and me in the months and years ahead. He thanked me for taking care of him, said he couldn't manage without me and hoped I would never leave him. As I said to him, where would I go and what would I do when I got there? Ralph was and always had been my only love, and I believed had become the God-given focus for my life at this time. I did not want it any other way.

There were good times. We had a couple of family barbecues and get-togethers and, while Ralph wasn't always entirely sure where he was, who was talking to him or why he was there, he was content. His grandchildren, increasingly unfamiliar to him, congregated around him, talked away, showed him photos on their phones and social media accounts and kept him supplied with juice and snacks. Ralph laughed and smiled his way through those evenings, and they were very special times that we can all look back on with great pleasure and thankfulness.

An early Christmas present

Over the years, we had often started to have conversations about Christmas in the month of October. With only me working and earning, October was when we accepted that there were only three pay cheques before Christmas (as I usually got December's pay before the 25th), and so that was the month when we began planning how we would save and allocate our funds to buy presents for family, friends and each other. However, in more recent years, these conversations had been somewhat one-sided, with me more or less telling him how much we would spend and on whom.

To my surprise, it was after Ralph came out of this particularly bad time in October 2017 that he initiated a conversation about Christmas – or rather, to be more accurate, about what I was going to get for Christmas. He went over and over what money he had, what I wanted and when we were going to get it. I tried to say we should wait until at least November to get our presents, but he got extremely agitated and said he wanted to get my presents now. For several mornings as I was getting him up, he said he wanted to get shaved, put his good trousers on, get a coordinating shirt and jumper and have his brown shoes on so that we could go out to get my presents. I thought he would forget with each morning but he didn't, and so eventually, for the first time ever in our marriage, we went out one October morning to buy my Christmas presents.

On the first shopping trip we bought a handbag. I picked one out, showed it to Ralph in the shop, took his wallet, paid for it, gave him back his wallet and showed him the receipt. When we got home, I then showed him where I had put the bag away, ready for Christmas. The next morning, as soon as Ralph was awake, he started again about getting my Christmas present and when we would get my handbag. I showed him the handbag put away and he was happy. The next morning again he asked about a handbag, had we got it, where was it and what else did I want? This was replayed every morning for a week. Then he stopped. When I asked him about Christmas, he said it was a bad time and he didn't want it. That worried me more than the previous days' repeated conversations about the handbag.

November began crisp and dry, more like December weather, and it enabled us to get out and about a fair bit. We enjoyed going out together to do some shopping, or rather me to do the shopping and Ralph to sit in the car until I returned. We even managed to enjoy the odd coffee out, depending on how stable he was on his feet. On days when we could do these small things, he seemed to relish feeling the air on his face and the breeze in his hair. Ralph loved putting on his heavier winter coat and especially his gloves. I kept them in the car and as soon as he got strapped in, he asked for his gloves. On a good day he could put them on himself, but usually he needed help as he would inevitably put them on the wrong hands or even put them on back to front, and then he would look at them quizzically, knowing that they were not right but unable to work out why.

While I was driving along, I would comment on the blue sky or scudding clouds. I would point out the leaves on the trees that had turned their beautiful autumnal colours and then show him the bare trees that had already lost theirs. I would tell him to look at the sheep in the fields, the cows grazing or lining up beside the hedges, and he would sometimes follow my pointed finger or look out of the window to see what I was talking about. However, he rarely responded, and often I didn't even know if he either heard me or understood what I was saying. Conversations were becoming one-way and passive. I spoke, Ralph listened; I asked questions, he just looked back at me without answering. He smiled his beautiful, simple, heartfelt smile. It was response enough.

An unforgettable Indian experience

When I left Nepal in January 1988, I decided to take a holiday in India before heading home. I planned to spend some time in Delhi and Goa with a mission friend who was also leaving Nepal at that time and returning to Germany. However, through a most peculiar set of unforeseen and bizarre circumstances, I ended up by myself in Delhi and, despite some understandable reservations, decided to continue with the planned trip. After a few days in Delhi seeing the sights, I flew to Goa and had an unforgettable two weeks there by myself. I discovered that when you are alone as a tourist in a strange place, you are more proactive and outgoing because you have to be, otherwise you would just sit in your hotel room all day. When you are by yourself, you have and do seek out more opportunities to meet people and go to places to fill your days. In retrospect, that trip to Goa showed me that solo holidays are not frightening but can actually be adventurous and exciting, as well as confidence-building and self-affirming.

One evening while in Goa, I went with some new friends I had met, who were staying in the same hotel as me, to a beach restaurant they had heard about. To call it a restaurant was somewhat generous, as it was basically just a few disparate tables abandoned on the beach above the tidemark and positioned underneath a rather precarious tarpaulin-style gazebo. There was a makeshift kitchen to one side of the tables that wouldn't have been passed by any environmental health officers in the UK, and a large bonfire to the other side, around which an assortment of locals and tourists were enjoying beers and a smoke, including, if my nostrils were to be believed, inhalations of a somewhat dubious genre. But that aside, I had a most memorable evening and without doubt one of the simplest yet best meals of my life. We dined on huge locally caught shrimp served with garlic butter and hunks of naan-like bread, all served family style with us all eating from shared platters.

After the meal, my new-found friends were intent on savouring the night, and it was obvious they intended to stay there for a few hours and enjoy the conversation and their nightcaps. However, I was tired so I decided to wander back to the hotel by myself, which meant walking along the beach around the bay for about half a mile.

As I approached the hotel, I passed some dhow-like boats draped with fishing nets and nearly jumped out of my skin when one of them just seemed to come to life and glide down the beach in front of me and heave itself into the sea. I realised, in fact, that three fishermen were propelling it into the water, and as I watched once the boat started to float in the seawater, they jumped into it and frantically paddled it over the crashing waves and into the sea proper. The sun was just going down and so I flopped onto the beach and watched as the boat headed out into the Arabian Sea.

I then had undoubtedly one of the most surreal experiences of my life. As I sat on the seashore, I watched the boat turn through ninety degrees and, as two of the fishermen paddled it across the sea, parallel with the shoreline, the third stood on the prow of the boat, threw his net into the water and then pulled it in, retrieving any fish from the net before repeatedly throwing it back in. The sun was setting, and as I watched the boat move along the surface of the sea and the sun move down towards the ocean rim, I realised I was about to see something truly magical.

For a fleeting second, I was witness to the most wonderful, amazing, incredible sight, the sort that posters and award-winning photographs are made of. A perfect picture, an amazing apparition and a sight of heart-wrenching beauty. As the sun finally hit the surface of the ocean in a red ball on the pink and golden horizon, the dhow skirted along the water and, by the freak that is nature, seemed to skim along the setting sun. The fisherman threw his net into the air just when the boat was in the centre of the ball, forming the most exquisite silhouette of the standing fisherman with his arms outstretched, his net hanging in the air and the boat in the centre of the setting sun. For me it was as if time stood still. I cried. I cried at the amazing sight I was witnessing, but I also cried because I was alone and I had no one to share this sight with. I realised that night, if I didn't already know, that true beauty is only fully appreciated when it is shared with another human being. Beauty has its zenith of fulfilment in being a shared experience, in being able to say, 'Isn't that beautiful?' to another soul; in being able to share with another human being a sight that is exquisite, beyond description and needs no definition or explanation.

The lonely life of a carer

As I became increasingly aware that our ability to share conversations and life experiences was becoming less and less, I'm afraid to say that I cried again. I cried that Ralph would never again say to me, 'Isn't that a wonderful sunset?' or, 'Did you see those beautiful clouds?' or comment on what a lovely dress I was wearing. I cried that I would never again be able to share what I saw as beautiful with Ralph, because he couldn't experience it with or without me. And I got angry again. Angry that all that I had once hoped for in our retirement years was crumbling around me, no matter how hard I tried to hold on to it. So much for all the things we were going to do, all the places we were going to see and all the time we would have together to do these things. Our hope for meaningful, shared experiences in the autumn and winter time of our lives here on earth was disintegrating around us and being washed away in the detritus of this disease. I felt that it was chipping away at us one moment, one experience and one opportunity at a time, relentlessly, progressively and completely.

Even simple pleasures that we used to share, like eating nice meals that I had cooked especially for us, were no longer possible. I always asked Ralph, and continue to do so, after we have eaten, if he enjoyed his meal. We had a game we used to play with new meals and dishes I cooked or when we ate out, where we would rank what we had eaten out of ten. I invariably asked him to do that if I had tried a new recipe, and our benchmark for having that new dish again was eight; if we scored the dish less than that, we didn't think it worth repeating. Now, at this stage on our 'D' journey, when I asked Ralph if he enjoyed his dinner or a new recipe I had tried, he just would say, 'Yes, thank you,' as if I was a waitress, and his ability to give a new dish a score out of ten had gone completely.

I realised that this lack of shared experience lessened both of our abilities to truly and fully experience beauty, wonder, mystery and, in real terms, delight. Once again, I was embittered and enraged at this 'D' life we were now forced to lead through no choice of our own. I was frustrated that even simple things such as sights and sounds could no longer be shared. It suddenly dawned on me that the single path that had begun when we married more than twenty-six years earlier was now beginning to permanently separate. It was like an iceberg splitting into pieces and being pulled apart by warm currents it was never meant to be in. This wretched 'D' journey we were forced to be on now was pulling us away from each other on different paths leading to different destinations.

For me, this time in our 'D' journey reinforced my increasingly confirmed belief and experience that dementia is a cruel, cruel disease. It not only forces an individual to walk along a lonely path into their own oblivion, away from the life they have previously known and into an existence of vacancy and nothingness, but it also forces those they love to walk a separate and different, never again to be shared path. Sadly, there is absolutely nothing either person can do to make those paths one again.

Dementia makes a mockery of marriage. Two don't become – or perhaps, more accurately, don't stay – as one. They drift away from each other, pulled apart by this hideous decayer of minds and dissolver of personality. Dementia splits and divides. It puts up barriers. It blocks hopes and dreams. It kills passion and desire and it replaces all that was once the very essence of a marriage with nothing, absolutely nothing.

I hated it afresh.

7

The Giant That Is Fear

I know that there are times in everyone's life when they experience worry or anxiety, but hopefully it is rare for an individual to experience outright terror, numbing dread or a fear that paralyses. It is easy to say that Christians, or indeed individuals of any faith, should not experience such fears, as we should believe that our lives are in the hands of God, or whatever greater being that we follow. However, the living-out of that belief is something that challenges people of all faiths and none.

We read in the Bible that 'perfect love drives out fear' (1 John 4:18). However, the reality for many of us is that every day we fear and plan for battles we will never be asked to fight, imagine situations that will never happen and live dreading what might or could happen to bring our world crashing down around us.

I have always been a glass-half-full type of person, as opposed to having a glass-half-empty approach to life. While there have been many occasions when I have been in difficult situations and been afraid, I am thankful that there have only been a couple of times when I have experienced true fear: once when I was caught up in a landslide when I worked in Papua New Guinea as a volunteer nutritionist for two years immediately after completing my degree, and on another occasion when I had a car accident in Northern Ireland.

Ralph, by contrast, has always been what I would describe as a 'worrier'. Indeed, I always joked that if there actually was nothing for him to worry about because everything in his or our lives seemed to be going well, he would worry about not having anything to worry about. Sometimes this worrying would consume him and he would become extremely fearful and anxious about the past, the present and the future. However, as November rolled on, I saw Ralph experience a level of fear that I had never seen him experience before. Even more concerning for me was the fact that, despite my presence with him, my love and my reassurances of my and God's love for him, his fear was not driven out but rather grew and deepened. I saw what fear, real fear, looked like close up in Ralph's eyes. I saw its effect on his health and I saw what impact it began to have on our relationship and our marriage.

It began with the shortening of the days and coincided with a couple of weeks of really bad zoned-out periods, so bad that I had further interactions with health and social services. It seemed to me that when the daylight started to wane earlier, Ralph started to become more and more unsettled earlier and earlier in the day. He became agitated, to put it mildly. He frequently wandered around the entire house, sitting in various rooms for a few seconds and then moving around from room to room, bed to bed, seat to seat. At dinner time he would not sit for any length of time to eat his dinner but would stand up and sit down repeatedly, eating mouthfuls of his meal in both positions. I even had to follow him around the house sometimes with a plateful of food and an outstretched fork to try to get him to eat.

When I asked Ralph if he was worried, he said he was, but when I asked him what he was worried about, he said he couldn't tell me. It was impossible to know whether he couldn't tell me or wouldn't tell me. As this behaviour progressed, he became totally fixated on me and on being close to me. When I left him lying down on top of our bed for a rest and said I was going to the kitchen to prepare food or do some ironing, it was only a matter of seconds until he had followed me and was standing at the kitchen door looking over at me as if he had seen a ghost. When I went out on my afternoons off, he was really unhappy, and when I came back he was often grumpy at least and angry at most that I had been away.

A couple of weeks into this pattern of behaviour, as Ralph was just beginning to settle down after an evening of wandering and agitation, he looked at me beside him on our bed and said, 'Are you going to leave me?' I stared at him in disbelief that he could ever in all seriousness ask me such a question. But I could see from his eyes and demeanour that he genuinely had been thinking about this possibility and that he was completely afraid that I would reply with a 'yes'. I, of course, said that I would never leave him, that I was here to stay and would always stay with him, and he accepted my reply on that occasion. But this was the start of this question being asked time and time again, day after day. So often was this question asked that I very quickly came to realise that this was the crux of Ralph's fear and agitation. He was completely terrified that I would leave him and that he would be alone.

Sometimes when Ralph was wandering around or getting up and down from the sofa or the bed, he would rock back and forth, drop his head and put his hands on it and start to mumble to himself. I hated to see him like this, stressed and distressed, but was powerless to reach him in this state, let alone help him. I would put my arms around him, hold him close and tell him time and time again that I was with him, that I wasn't leaving him and that I loved him. On one occasion after I had told him this several times, Ralph looked at me and said, 'Why me? Why did I get like this?' and he was almost in tears as he bowed his head and said, 'Too much to bear, too much to bear.' It took hours sometimes for him to settle, and then mercifully he became so exhausted after all the stress he had been through that he put his head back on the pillow and slept. I could only hope that his sleep was peaceful and restful and that the fears subsided, even if they did not disappear completely.

Fear that corrodes

What makes us truly fear something, anything, known or unknown? Perhaps it is the latter, fear of the unknown, that we fear the most. To cope with what we don't know, we might fantasise, or sometimes make up possible or probable scenarios that may enable us to cope with what might happen. Or perhaps it is the former, the fear of the known. We replay in our minds what happened in a particular situation. We remember what we or someone else did or said, and we can become consumed and even distressed by the effect this had on us as we relive it. If we have to face those circumstances or individuals again, this distress can then progress into a sense of fear that can affect us physically, mentally and emotionally.

As we get older and have years of life experience behind us, we often know only too well that evil can appear to triumph in our world, that bad things do happen to good people and that the Christian life is not a bed of roses but rather a constant fight against the wiles of the devil and his desire to pull us away from God. However, even though we accept and acknowledge this, when we have to face the challenge of such 'bad' things happening in our lives, we can find ourselves extremely fearful. This fear may even develop to the point where we can be deeply and sometimes irreparably affected or damaged by it.

To face fear, deal with it, overcome it and survive it is hard enough for anyone of sound mind and body to cope with, but to face it with a diagnosis of dementia must be life-sapping. I could see the fear eat Ralph up from the inside out. He appeared to get smaller and smaller. He seemed increasingly frail and was sinking into himself as this incredible burden of his fear that I would leave him and his realisation of the deterioration in his mental state weighed more and more heavily on his shoulders. His appetite began to fail, he spent more time in bed and it became difficult to get him to go out for a coffee or even to sit in the car while I ran around the town and did a few calls. He was almost constantly unsettled, stared at me with huge unblinking eyes for minutes at a time and then often sighed and looked as if he was going to burst into tears. Occasionally, when he was able to, he would say things like, 'I'm not well,' or, 'What's going to become of me?' and always somewhere in such conversations the same question would surface: 'Are you going to leave me?'

Fear not

It has always been a great source of encouragement to me that the Bible so often speaks of fear or of being afraid in the form of a negative command. Namely, it admonishes fear and frequently instructs us not to fear or be troubled, in strong if not forceful words.[6] If we feel afraid, the book of Psalms is where we can find so many verses that tell us not to fear, because God is with us and will deliver us from all that we are anxious about.[7] I have found great comfort in this book in times past and present when my heart has been troubled.

But equally, it has always been a source of great encouragement to me that in the Bible we read stories of weakness turned to strength. The apostle Peter succumbed to his fear for a time (Matthew 26:69-75), yet was graciously restored (John 21:15-19) and went on to become a great leader in the first-century Church. In the Old Testament, the patriarch Abram (Abraham) was afraid, and lied (Genesis 12:10-13, 19). Moses, too, was

---

[6] Isaiah 41:10; Matthew 10:31; Mark 5:36.
[7] Psalm 27:1; Psalm 56:3; Psalm 91:5.

fearful and ran away (Exodus 2:14-15). Then there is the story of Gideon in Judges 6–8, and of how God provided sufficient grace and strength for him to overcome his fears.

Despite such weaknesses, God used His children in the fulfilment of His will, and can do the same for us (2 Corinthians 12:9). I like to think that these biblical stories are included in God's Word to remind us in our generation that the victory over fear and over the circumstances that engender it in our lives is through God's strength that is freely available to us all, weak and frail as we are in such experiences.

I think again of Peter, who had enough faith in his Lord to get out of the boat and stand on the water and take those first steps, but once fear kicked in and he took his eyes off his Lord, he sank (Matthew 14:28-31). Or Elijah, the Old Testament prophet who fled in fear of his life under the persecution of Jezebel (1 Kings 18–19) but went on to mightily serve God.

By contrast, fear can also have the effect on us that it had on Joshua, the successor to Moses, who when he heard the words God had for him, absolutely believed them:

> Have I not commanded you? Be strong and courageous. Do not be afraid; do not be discouraged, for the LORD your God will be with you wherever you go.
> *Joshua 1:9*

He then set out to fight the battles and win the victories that Moses never could. Fear can immobilise us into inactivity or make us sink into physical, mental, emotional or physical depths, like Peter. However, it can also, through God's grace and strength, be the stimulus for us to win battles we would never have willingly chosen to fight, and in the winning of which we will be assured and reassured that we are in the centre of His will.

One night, after a particularly bad evening of fear-driven agitation, I got Ralph to lie on the bed beside me and picked up his Bible. It opened at a page that he had dog-eared and I saw a passage that was underlined, no doubt at a time in his life when it spoke directly to him: 'In thee, O LORD, do I put my trust' (Psalm 31:1, AKJV). I continued to read the rest of the psalm and stopped when I read the first line of verse 15: 'My times are in thy hand'.

I said to Ralph, who was lying beside me with his eyes closed, 'Isn't that wonderful, that our times are in God's hands and that we can put our trust in Him?' He was silent, but I told him again how wonderful it was to know that God has our times in His hands. Then I read the two verses to him again. I put the Bible down and said nothing more but just left it there.

From then on, whenever Ralph was agitated for a time, I read passages of the Bible and hymns from his *Believers Hymn Book* to him, and it was amazing how they calmed him, if only for a few minutes. As I read, he stared straight ahead but was quiet and unmoving, focusing his attention on my voice, if not the words I was saying. After I ended the readings, I always made a few comments, such as, 'Wasn't that lovely?', 'Isn't it wonderful to know that God hears us... loves you... is with us... knows what we are going through?' Sometimes he would reply with a simple 'yes', but mostly he would just be silent. It didn't stop the fear coming back later or the next night, but for a few seconds or a few minutes he found peace, reassurance and calmness in God's Word and Christian verse.

Strength for the way

It was through reinstating this much-needed practice of reading and praying together again that I found a renewed appreciation for previously known psalms and well-known hymns with old-fashioned phrases that had been written in bygone times but contained such epoch-transcending truths. Some of the hymns I read seemed to have been written just for Ralph at this time, and one I came back to during those fear-ridden nights was 'Safe in the Arms of Jesus'. Some lines in the second verse were so apt:

> Safe in the arms of Jesus,
> Safe from corroding care,
> Safe from the world's temptations,
> Sin cannot harm me there.
> Free from the blight of sorrow,
> Free from my doubts and fears;
> Only a few more trials,
> Only a few more tears.[8]

I found myself being so thankful for men and women with the God-given gift of writing words and tunes that encourage and inspire their own and countless future

---

[8] Fanny Crosby (1820–1915), 'Safe in the Arms of Jesus', *Believers Hymn Book* (Kilmarnock: John Ritchie Ltd, 2008), 243. Revised edition. Public domain.

generations of Christians in their faith. I read Ralph words of encouragement from old hymns and choruses he would have been familiar with, written years ago and in different times to people of fragile faith or none; written for people who were fearful of life and living and to people uncertain of their eternal future. The old-fashioned words like 'covenant' and 'redemption', 'assurance' and 'consecration' coupled with concepts of eternal certainty, divine will and human frailty were read to him and for him primarily. However, they also challenged and encouraged me at this time to want to know and experience God more with us as we travelled along with Him on this 'D' journey.

Would we have chosen this as part of our shared journey? Absolutely not. Ralph may have got the dementia, but I became more aware that what I often think of as my individual Christian journey was not a solitary trek but rather a shared journey.

Our marriage journey was a united one and wherever this 'D' journey section of it was leading us, we were on it together and on it for life. The marriage vows Ralph and I took were real and visionary and the covenant we began more than twenty-six years earlier was now reaping its fulfilment in the reality of living them out. The sanctity and glory of the marriage begun in that ceremony all those years ago in a country church in Northern Ireland could easily have been degraded and eroded by this diagnosis. But, glory be to God, I realised it hadn't been and that what Ralph and I were experiencing now in this time of our marriage was the real meaning of living out those vows each and every day.

Shortly after we were married, Ralph said to me one evening that he thought people were often more in love with the idea of being married than the reality of living it. I believe he was right. The reality is tough as you both set off on a journey together. You don't know the destination. You certainly don't know long it will take to get there, and you don't know what will happen to you individually or together along the way. It's the not knowing that makes a marriage a marriage. If you had known what was ahead, you may never have started it. But the covenant that is marriage means that for those who truly believe their marriage vows, having started it you can't stop it, and the marriage will run its course. For some, sadly it ends with betrayal, for others with disease, and regrettably, in today's society for many it peters out with disillusionment. Hopefully for many, though, it is a lifelong journey of sharing, giving and receiving. Its ultimate end comes with the death of one partner, but even then it is not truly over, for its influence will transcend death and exert its impact on the remaining partner for the rest of their life.

Dementia had changed one human half of Ralph's and my marriage covenant irreparably, both physically and spiritually in the way he had deteriorated over these past years and year. However, it had also changed the other half of it too. It had changed me. Our covenant was still intact, our marriage vows current and the previous years spent together a wonderful blessing. But the months or years ahead? In reality, they were no different from the way it was for anyone setting out on a marriage journey today. The road ahead of us was, in the main, unknown and uncertain. However, in the midst of it all, one thing was undeniable: it was still a shared journey. A journey that would not peter out but run its full course and reach its ultimate goal in a love partnership that would of course one day reach its earthly end, but would then be transformed from this world's understanding of the meaning of marriage into an eternal relationship in heaven (Matthew 22:23-32).

Covenant love, sacrificial love and, above all, eternal love.

8

Joy in Our World

God is so good; despite all the zoned-out times he experienced in November, Ralph came back to me and to the family for Christmas.

I had begun to think that he wouldn't even make Christmas, he was physically so frail. Mentally he was so far away from us all and totally unable to connect with me, let alone anyone else, for the four weeks prior to it. Amazingly, however, just a few days before the big day, he came back from wherever he had been and reconnected with us all.

There had been a pattern to our Christmases over previous years that had come to symbolise what the Christmas season meant for us – places to be and people to see and just the two of us together for Christmas lunch. Then we usually headed out later in the day to join some of the family for a get-together in one of their homes. To my great surprise and joy, we were able to live out most of that pattern once again this Christmas. We visited family before and after the big day. We ate party food and we sat on the couch and watched all the repeats on television. We had a simple lunch on Christmas Day of stuffed roast chicken and his beloved sherry trifle for dessert. We looked into, not past, each other's eyes and we found a happiness that had been absent for months.

Needless to say, all the family were also so happy to see him like this again. Oh, he still didn't know them all the time, and he didn't always appreciate where he was and who he was with, but he was content to be with them. Ralph enjoyed their company in his own way, which was expressed in his ubiquitous quiet manner and smiling face.

Blessings come in so many shapes and forms. In previous years, blessings at Christmas had come in the giving of expensive presents between us both, and lots of lavish entertaining which we shared with others. I would spend hours in the kitchen producing meals worthy of the chefs whose recipes I took delight in trying to emulate. There were also times when we went away for a short break after the big day, or went up to the north coast of Northern Ireland, and we were so blessed to have those times and the resources to enable them to happen. But there are periods in all our lives when blessings are very simple and, by some standards, insignificant. In societal worth or monetary value terms, we would be hard-pressed to justify them as blessings in the sense that our materialistic world would understand, but in certain situations, they really are.

Blessings at Christmas

When I was living in Nepal during that three-year period in the mid-1980s, there were quite a few Northern Irish missionaries working with the mission I was placed there with. One Christmas, an Ulster family had a visit from a family member who, in an inspired gesture, brought out a full box of a well-known brand of cheese and onion potato crisps, and a packet was sent to every Northern Irish missionary in Nepal as a Christmas present. For those of us who were based in mission stations far from the beaten track, let alone a bus route, porters were employed to carry essential supplies and post to us on a weekly basis. That Christmas season I well remember a very squashed and flattened packet of crisps arriving in the porter's basket at our little house in the middle hills of Nepal. I remember savouring the crisps and even licking the plastic bag to get every last vestige of the familiar flavour that I could. That bag of crisps was what I would describe as a real blessing to me that Christmas. To some it might have been described as a poor excuse for a Christmas present, but to all of us who received an 'insignificant' bag of crushed crisps, it was a special blessing that triggered tastes, smells, sounds and experiences of home that brought us such joy.

The real blessing of Ralph coming out of such a prolonged zoned-out state as he had been in and returning to me for this Christmas was that he was truly with me. We could be a couple again, sharing experiences and talking rationally about things. I knew that if his health were to deteriorate as much in the coming year as it had in the past one, this would probably be the last Christmas when there was any real connection between us, and I was determined not to miss or waste a moment of it. I knew that to have this connection with him this Christmas was special and, like the remembered savouriness of that packet of crisps all those years ago, would create joyous memories that I would always have and could always treasure.

In particular, I cherished one special memory of this Christmas in 2017 which I could call on when Ralph retreated into his shrinking world again and from which I feared, one day, he would never emerge.

Each Christmas we have a family party before Christmas in one of our homes for however many of us can get together. We all bring food and have a pot-luck of casseroles and slow cooker dishes followed by a delight of desserts. Up until a day before the event that year, I was not at all sure that we would be able to go; if Ralph had been in a severe zoned-out state comparable to the one he experienced in late October, when he had a urinary tract infection, I could not have taken him. However, to my great joy, we did manage to get to it. Even though on the day of the party, Ralph was in a much better place mentally, I was concerned that the crowd of us all together, with the noise and excitement of children and adults, would be too much for him.

To try to protect him, I had arranged with Lynda, whose house the party was being held in, that Ralph could sit in one of her sitting rooms away from the kitchen where everyone normally congregated. In that way he could be in a calmer and quieter place, and individuals could go to him and chat with him on a one-to-one basis. That plan should have worked very well, except when we arrived at the house, I discovered that there happened to be a football match on that night and the television in the room where he was to sit was the one that all the guys wanted to watch the match on. Ralph had never really liked football, always preferring rugby. That night, however, he sat there entranced with children, sons-in-law, grandsons and co-father-in-law. They were all watching the match and actively rooting for and cheering on their side, and it soon became apparent that he was totally transfixed and engaged by it all.

All the guys from every generation in that room kept an eye on Ralph, and they included him in their comments on the match. I could hear some of his grandsons shouting, 'Did you see that, Pop?' from the kitchen where I was with the girls, and could also hear some of the others drawing his attention to their interpretation of the referee's handling of the game. They also kept him supplied with drinks and snacks on the little table Lynda had put beside his chair. I went in to check on him a couple of times, and on one occasion I arrived just as their team scored a goal. There was an enormous cheer and a great thumping of chairs and Ralph just looked up at me and smiled the biggest smile I had seen in ages – more, I think, at the antics of his fellow watchers than at the goal that had just been scored. I could see in that moment that he was so happy; that he felt included, even if he didn't fully understand what was going on. To anyone else in that room, it was just a typical Friday night; a room full of men watching other men kick a ball around a muddy pitch and getting overexcited about it. But to me, it was such a blessing to see Ralph taking part in a normal family event and, more than that, happy in a way he hadn't been for a long time.

Joy and happiness

In the quiet, dark days between Christmas and the New Year, we settled back into our normal routine and had good times together. I thought about the time of year we were in and what it meant to our world. Joy at the birth of a baby and the gift that it was to all humanity, albeit unrecognised by the world at that time.

Joy, for me, means experiencing feelings of happiness and pleasure; it makes me feel glad and content. It can be fleeting, like the pleasure we experience when eating a much-loved food, or it can be long-lasting, like the contentment we experience when we know that we are loved unconditionally by a parent, a friend or a partner. We may not always feel joyful about the circumstances we are experiencing, but through God's grace, we can know joy *in* them; in fact, James 1:2 tells us to 'consider it ... joy' when we go through trials.

Joy, when best experienced, is both an internal and an external emotion. We feel joy inside ourselves and, when we do, we express it by smiling or laughing, or with a contentment that is obvious in our demeanour. When we are joyful, it is impossible for others around us not to realise this. Our joy can be infectious, with those who see it in us then uplifted and made happy themselves. They smile back at us, they laugh with us, they note our contentment and sometimes express that they wish they could find it in their lives.

Happiness, as an expression of joy, is something that many of us strive to achieve in this world, but so often it is transient and elusive and we must make do with the small morsels we get. With the benefit of hindsight, we can look back at times in our lives when we experienced real and lasting joy, in family, in friends, in personal and career achievements and in love, and that experience of joy was even more meaningful because it was shared. If we are fortunate, such joy can engender a feeling of belonging, is fulfilling personally and in the company of others, and is satisfying in the broadest sense of the word. But it is also true that sometimes a memory of such joy can be a sharp and perhaps even painful reminder of a previous happier time.

Joy at Christmas was something ingrained into me from childhood. From the time I could stand up with the Sunday school choir, I sang about joy coming into our world in the form of the infant Jesus, and about those who were part of that first Christmas story. I remember singing carols that spoke of joy, triumph and peace, and always knew within my being that Christmas was essentially a happy time, as I understood being happy back then. There were family get-togethers, presents in abundance and special food and goodies. Everyone seemed happy, and Christmas was always a longed-for occasion and much missed when it was over. A very special time.

By contrast, Ralph never really liked Christmas as a season. I never got to the bottom of why that was, and now I never will. He tolerated it, is possibly the best way I could put it. I am sure that Ralph did experience happiness and pleasure in all the activities he and we had enjoyed over the years we were able to fully celebrate it together, but he was always glad when Christmas was over. His attitude to this time of the year always reminded me that perhaps for him and for so many people, Christmas is not a time of joy, but rather of sadness. Sadness at missing loved ones, or sadness at another year lived and the awareness of another year less to live, or perhaps sadness at a lack of happiness in one's life at a time when everyone else seems to be experiencing ecstatic and exuberant joy. I wondered if Ralph's mere tolerance of Christmas was because of some previous experience that was painful or elicited sadness, and that the current season evoked those memories.

Lost and found joys

I thought about Naomi in the book of Ruth in the Bible. She, along with her husband and two sons, had left their home in Bethlehem in difficult times and travelled, like so many people do today, to try to find a better life in a new country. At first, they seemed to manage this, her beloved sons even marrying local girls. Happy times, I'm sure. Then tragedy struck. First her husband and then her two sons died. Joy experienced and then gone. In that male-dominated world, no doubt the future seemed bleak and frightening for the three now-single women who had been widowed so suddenly, and so Naomi decided to return to the land of her birth. Perhaps she wanted to return to a place where she had found happiness before and leave a place that was now devoid of any joy for her, and of which she had only bitter memories. In a well-known passage, we learn how Ruth's persistence in wanting to remain with her mother-in-law meant that Naomi did not return to her homeland alone, but with one of her daughters-in-law by her side (Ruth 1:14-19.)

When they arrived back in Bethlehem, Naomi met up with some former neighbours, who possibly reminded her of the joy and happiness she had once had, and in a fit of pique she told them:

> Don't call me Naomi … Call me Mara, because the Almighty has made my life very bitter. I went away full, but the LORD has brought me back empty.
> *Ruth 1:20-21*

The joy in her life had long gone and her planned change of name makes me think that she had no hope that it would ever return. However, God's plans were in motion and, by a wonderful set of divine circumstances Ruth, a daughter-in-law who probably up to that point had been a daily reminder of Naomi's losses, became the route by which joy came back into Naomi's life.

I often wonder if she ever asked her neighbours to change the name they called her back to Naomi? I hope so. I hope it was *Naomi* who dandled Ruth and Boaz's son on her knee and rediscovered her lost joy. That it was *Naomi* who hopefully was given an insight that the messianic dynasty that started with Adam and ended with Jesus Christ included Ruth, and by association included her. Joy personified in Naomi. Sadness in Mara. Hope in Naomi. Bitterness in Mara. Joy and sadness, like two sides of the one coin, or light in comparison to darkness or hope compared to bitterness. One difficult to quantify without the other as a reference.

For some reason when I think about Naomi and her change of name to Mara, I always think of horseradish sauce, that strong, piquant condiment that is served most often with roast beef. If you taste horseradish by itself on the end of a fork or spoon, it will bring tears to your eyes and constrict your throat. However, a little dabbed on the end of a forkful of prime roast beef totally enhances the flavour, so that you taste the sweetness of the beef in a way not possible without it. It takes the piquancy of the sauce to make you realise how wonderfully sweet and succulent the beef tastes. I think that it took Mara's grief at the loss of one family to enable Naomi to find true happiness again in a new family and a renewed life.

As the daylight hours began to lengthen even by a few minutes each day, I felt lightened and brightened by the experiences of this particular Christmas. Was it the same as those Christmases of years before, where we spent so much money on material gifts? Were the memories we would have of it comparable to my recollections of the fabulous meals, excessive eating and late nights of chatting and 'craic'[9] we had previously enjoyed? Did it remind me of those happy Christmas times of my childhood when everything was magical and shiny and glittering and joyful and triumphant? Or was it perhaps more akin to what I thought might be Ralph's long-held mere tolerance of the season, in that the joys of this current Christmas might only serve to remind me of happier times in the past?

---

[9] 'Craic' is a common expression in Northern Ireland that we use to say we are having a really good time.

Joy for me now – and I hoped that it was the same for Ralph, though he was unable to express it – was in the being, not the getting. It was in accepting that I was the half, not the whole. Joy for me was being with Ralph, where he was, sharing how he was in the present. While knowing that it might not always be so, joy, real joy, could be experienced in the here and now. Of course, there were and would be bitter times, fearful times and sad times ahead for both of us. But I realised that for Ralph at this point in his life, his obsession with having me near him and never wanting me out of his sight was what he now considered joy. Likewise, his being with people who affirmed him, spent time with him, brought him food and included him in their activities were truly happy, joyful experiences. By contrast, my absence from his presence meant for him an absence of joy in his now life and caused him fear and distress.

For me, being with Ralph was truly my joy, and while I could be bitter at the loss of meaningful time I had with him owing to this 'D' life we were living, in a peculiar way it enabled me to fully appreciate what we had known in the past and could experience again in each and every real moment we shared together.

The reality for Ralph and for me at this stage of our 'D' journey was that every little, seemingly insignificant joy we had together was enhanced because of the difficult, somewhat bitter times we had experienced and would undoubtedly experience in the future as we travelled on together. But having acknowledged that, we could accept that it only took a little of the bitter experiences to help us both, in our own ways, to appreciate how blessed we were with the joys we now had, and how important it was to savour every precious one while we could.

Our glass was more than half full; it was brimming and running over, and I knew it would always be so if I could just see it.

9

A New Year Begins

Neither of us was ever really into making New Year's resolutions. I could never see the point of committing to something just because of a particular date on the calendar, but did completely understand the need from time to time to commit to a different way of living or lifestyle. There were a number of times, throughout any one year and over several years in our married life, when Ralph and I did commit to changing our diet, increasing our exercise routine, supporting a particular individual or charity, or planned to spend less time watching television and more time with each other.

However, for me, this particular New Year seemed to accentuate the need to completely ignore as irrelevant the usual mantra for self-imposed change associated with 1st January. I was just coping where I was. The thought of actually choosing to making any changes in my life, apart from the ones that were foisted on me daily, was too exhausting to contemplate.

Ralph and I spent New Year's Eve like any other Sunday night in 2017, sitting at the fireside after a lazy and quiet day, watching a little television and then heading to our bedroom at around 7.30. He had changed into his pyjamas and took his night-time medication as usual around eight o'clock, and shortly afterwards was out for the count. I decided that I would stay up to see the New Year in and lie on the top of the bed beside him, watching television while he slept. However, by the time 10.30 came, I could see no point in staying up by myself and, as I was tired after a wearying few days, I turned the light off and 2018 slipped into our home all by itself, unmarked and unnoticed. There seemed nothing either of us wanted to celebrate or commend about this particular night, let alone the year passing and, if truth be told, I was glad to see the back of it.

Psalm 139 has always been a favourite of mine. There is so much in it that is personal and individually inspiring, yet also challenging and demanding. It was the psalm that challenged me to seek God's will in serving him abroad and resulted in me working in Nepal for three years. It was the psalm that I turned to when I was diagnosed with cancer and found assurance that God knew all about it and would be with me in it, so I could trust Him through it. It is also the psalm that always reminds me of how intimately God loves me, no matter where I am, what I'm doing or what I have done. There is a wonderful verse in it that says, 'I praise you because I am fearfully and wonderfully made' (Psalm 139:14). As I reread the psalm at this time, I was struck by the thought that this might include the concept of being 'fearfully and wonderfully' *continuously* 'made'. Our bodies are constantly being remade, with every cell in our bodies on a continuous renewal cycle. Our bodies grow and regenerate throughout our lives, and God's creator hand directs and oversees all those changes at cellular, whole-body and mind levels.

Just as everybody ages and as a consequence of that process changes internally and externally, so I realised afresh that Ralph's body had a dual aspect of change. He was undergoing the normal ageing process that anyone does, as he was well into his eighth decade, but he was also undergoing internal physiological and cerebral changes and experiencing their external consequences as a result of his dementia. I found this aspect of his changing frustrating and confusing. Over the previous months, when changes had occurred in his physical or mental health, I was sometimes hard pressed to work out whether they were as a result of the natural ageing process, his dementia, or something else going on that required medical intervention. It was all too easy for me – and, if I'm honest, for others – to put any negative changes or new symptoms that he exhibited down to his dementia and not consider other causes. Just because he had dementia did not mean that he couldn't develop a heart problem, get the flu or a stomach bug, or have a bad day and get depressed or angry at something.

Nature or nurture?

Immediately after Ralph's diagnosis, believing that knowledge is power, I went on to the internet and trawled everything I could find on dementia and, as usual when you do that, ended up with knowledge overload and complete saturation of facts, figures and conjecture. Since his diagnosis, from time to time as he behaved in different ways from what I knew or expected, I had often wondered about the physiology, the chemistry and the neurology of dementia in its various forms. I never believed that I had the intellect myself to be able to even partially understand the vastness of both the complexity and minutiae of the human body, never mind the brain. However, my general science background gave me enough understanding to appreciate the genius and intellect of medical doctors, postgraduate scientists and researchers whose lives were dedicated to exploring the abyss and heights of the well and not-so-well human body and mind, particularly in relation to the various diseases classified within the dementia portfolio.

It was at this time, early 2018, that I recognised, to my surprise, my lack of continued interest in the physiological and neurological aspects of Ralph's changing symptoms and disease. I was accepting, not questioning, of his condition now, and how it impacted his life and living. I had never given any serious thought as to why Ralph, as opposed to the individuals or population groups thought to be at higher risk of developing the disease as described in the dementia studies and articles I had previously read, had developed it. Was there anything in his or our lifestyles that had increased the risk for him of developing the mixed dementia he had been diagnosed with? Had anything he or we had done or not done caused it, contributed to it or exacerbated it? Was it down to nature or nurture? Fate or circumstance? Divine providence or personal failures? What should or could we do about that now? Was it worthwhile making any changes to our diet or lifestyle now, or was it better just to be accepting of where we were and let nature take its course along the road we had been travelling up to this point and were continuing on?

I began to concern myself with why, if Ralph was 'fearfully and wonderfully made', as the psalmist suggests, he had been 'fearfully and wonderfully made' this way. How could it ever be part of God's plan for Ralph, as one of His creations, to slowly degenerate over the years until he was completely unmade from the man that he had been? Surely God would not unpick and unravel Ralph until he no longer bore any resemblance to how God created him? Even though I understood that this happened to Ralph as a consequence of the Fall (Genesis 3), I felt quite aggrieved at a God who could allow it to happen to someone I cared about so much. I thought that if Ralph had been diagnosed with a cancer or a heart condition, perhaps I would have accepted it better or more readily. While physically he might have become frail and weak in a similar way to his current and most likely future state of health, I would still have had the essence of him with me. Then I realised that I was guilty of ranking his diagnosis with other life-limiting diseases and conditions and, on this scale, he was always going to come up short with his incurable duet of dementia syndromes.

I took myself back to the internet and read and reread strategies, plans and scholarly and not-so-scholarly articles on the subject. I read again about this progressive, degenerative and irreversible quiver of diseases, more common in people more than sixty-five years of age, with the estimated incidence in the UK being one in fourteen people more than sixty-five years of age and one in six people more than eighty years of age. I read much discussion but few definitive conclusions on specific measures that might help to prevent the disease, with the consensus only on advising people to follow general lifestyle guidance for the population, including healthy eating, taking more exercise, not smoking and moderating alcohol intake. Some strategies and studies also mentioned the importance of avoiding and tackling loneliness and social isolation and cognitive stimulation, like doing puzzles or learning a new language in preventing the disease.[10]

Then, of course, there were the dementia strategies at national and regional level with their plethora of recommendations, action plans, goals and often detailed performance measures by which progress, whatever that was defined as, could be assessed. Interestingly, it was less common to find any reports on the implementation of those action plans or any assessments of progress towards the goals so boldly written in the summaries of these pristine strategies which most likely adorn the bookshelves of many a service provider. Then there were additional reports and lobbying articles from charities, individuals and interested bodies outlining their suggestions and proposals for research, action and change. The literature and articles on dementia were

_____

[10] Public Health England, 'Health matters: midlife approaches to reduce dementia risk' (March 2016), www.gov.uk/government/publications/health-matters-midlife-approaches-to-reduce-dementia-risk/ (Accessed 11th January 2021).

breath-taking in their range and depth, but the more I read, the harder I found it to directly relate them to Ralph or to me.

He was a lifelong non-smoker. Tick. He never drank alcohol. Tick. He really didn't care much for red meat, preferring fish and chicken. Tick. He wasn't great at taking exercise. He did not have much social interaction with others outside the family, and throughout his life had struggled with depression and anxiety disorders, receiving medication for these. No ticks. We did have a healthy diet and I always considered it one of my greatest successes to have taken the man I married, who had a very limited palate and a penchant for double-layer pastry pies, and gradually encourage him to become a more discerning amateur gourmet and healthy eater. Ralph loved home cooking, particularly mine, and especially homemade soups, stews and casseroles. He disliked desserts that were overly sweet, his favourite pudding being apple crumble and custard. Neither of us really liked chocolate, so we rarely had sweets in the house, and if we received any for Christmas we usually gave them away.

So, did I think on reflection that there was anything in our history that might have given rise to this 'D' life we were now experiencing, anything that had contributed to it or increased its risk? Genuinely, as I thought about it, I didn't think so. Ralph had been careful about his body, about what he put into it, how he treated it, and I was certainly careful about what we both had eaten. Not that that was ever because of a desire to prevent dementia, but rather to follow the general healthy eating guidelines recommended for the population. Of course, there were things which in hindsight we might have pursued more vigorously, such as more physical or brain exercise. But in general, I felt we both had lifestyles in the past and were continuing with them now that, as I compared us to what I had read in my internet perusals, were supportive of what was purported in the literature as being preventative or curative to a diagnosis or experience of dementia.

So logically, the next step was to ask myself whether there was anything we should or could change about our lifestyle now in light of both what was proposed if not accepted best practice in dementia research. As I reflected on that, the short answer was no. I confirmed in my mind that our diet was healthy and that there were no substances that he should avoid or actively include more of. He had more social interaction now than when I was working, and while his physical health precluded him from taking long walks, we did still get out and about when opportunities arose. As far as he could walk, even if it was only from the house to the car or, when he was able, from the car to the inside of a coffee shop, we did that two or three times each week. He took his medication for the Alzheimer's part of his mixed dementia and he took other tablets to lessen the impact of other conditions on it. Could we benefit from more social interaction? Possibly. Could I encourage him to do puzzles, or read a newspaper or a book? He had never done these things before, so how useful would it be for him to do them now? Were these rationalisations about his lifestyle just me being lazy and complacent about him and not pushing him more assertively to proactively engage in his lifestyle at this time?

I remembered decades earlier giving a healthy eating talk to a group of health and social care service providers. After my input, as usual in these situations, there was an allotted time for questions. One member of the audience asked me a specific question about a client of hers who had an eating pattern she thought very unhealthy in a number of aspects. This man, who lived alone in the country, began each day with two raw duck eggs beaten into a pint of unpasteurised raw milk. As the man was a semi-retired farmer, in the sense that farmers never really retire, he had ducks and cows on the farm and had used their produce all his life. The lady was concerned not just about the negative nutritional aspects of this concoction, but also about its bacteriological implications. In response to her question, I asked the lady what age her client was, and she replied that he was eighty-eight. After a collective intake of breath and chuckling from the audience, my response was that if he had lived to the age of eighty-eight on a breakfast of raw milk and uncooked duck eggs, was there really any justification in encouraging him to change his eating pattern now? I would still stand by that answer. There is more to food than nutrients, more to life than years and more to personal fulfilment and pleasure than scientific reasoning can measure.

Happiness and contentment

I then asked myself the questions that I had been avoiding in all of this internet trawling, scientific exploration and lifestyle questioning. Was Ralph happy in his life now? Did he live a contented life? Would he change anything in his life right now if he could? If I were to change anything in our shared lifestyle that affected his quality of life, how would he or how would I know that any resulting change was for the better – whatever 'for the better' would mean for Ralph? I thought about that for days, watching him as he struggled, as he smiled and laughed and as he left me in his zoned-out days. What was happiness for him in his life and lifestyle now, and how could he and I recognise and improve it? I came to accept that our individual and shared happiness was different from what we had had in years past, but that there was still individual and shared happiness for us both in the lifestyle that we had developed over the years and were now living. We were just using different measuring techniques to assess whether it was a happy and contented lifestyle for us individually and together. We would never be able to prove beyond scientific reason or doubt that it was the correct lifestyle for us right now on our 'D' journey, but equally we couldn't or didn't need to prove that it wasn't.

Ralph smiled more now than I had ever known him to do. I loved to see him smile, and so did others. He laughed, sometimes a childlike laugh that replaced words that would not come to him, but it was still a happy laugh. For the most part he enjoyed his food. He enjoyed the soft feel of his throw on the bed. He watched the logs burn on the fire and smiled when they crackled. Of course, in the zoned-out times he didn't smile or laugh, but when he came out of those states, I was so happy that increasingly he had no memory of ever being in them. The bad times were never remembered by Ralph and that in itself was happiness to me. I would have been broken-hearted if he remembered the incontinence, the inability to feed himself, or to put his arms into his sweater, or to know how to sit down on a chair. Did I want to try to improve his memory of and in those situations? Absolutely not. Ralph lived in the moment with me and that moment was a happy one. We were happy together now and that was all that truly mattered.

I went back to Psalm 139 and this time it was another verse that stopped me in my tracks.

> All the days ordained for me were written in
> your book
> before one of them came to be.
> *Psalm 139:16*

God knew exactly what had lain ahead for Ralph and me as we had set off on this 'D' journey together. He had shaped me to cope with all that it had brought already and would undoubtedly bring to us both in the future, and He had mercifully spared Ralph painful memories of difficult times he experienced along the way.

God knew that we would walk this way together, and at this time on our journey I had a renewed sense that His grace would be sufficient for us, both now and in the days to come.

10
Asking for Help

In the first six months after I retired from work in 2015, in many respects Ralph and I had a really lovely time getting out and about and enjoying quality time together. This was exactly what I had hoped for in my retirement. But as I looked back, what shocked me was how much Ralph physically and mentally deteriorated in that time. It was as if his body and mind just breathed a huge sigh of relief that I was permanently home with him, and he let all his control and determination to manage his own life and health go. I realised very quickly in those first few weeks and months of my time with Ralph just how much he must have been struggling to cope on his own, what tremendous inner strength and resilience he had drawn upon to manage those last weeks I worked, as he spent every day waiting for me to come home. I could almost see him physically droop with the relief of not having to fight through each lonely day and being able to pass the baton of managing his life on to me.

Ralph had a very small circle of friends when I met him. Given the challenges that a second marriage meant for him and the challenge of being a second wife brought to me, we were careful about sharing details of our lives before we met or of bringing aspects of those individual and very different lives into our marriage. While we were going out with each other, we had made an agreement not to ask each other personal questions about our lives and relationships before we met, with each of us sharing with the other only what we wished to about those times. We wanted to start afresh so that our relationships, friends and memories were jointly made and shared. Of course, there were exceptions with extended family and a couple of lifelong friends of his who became shared friends for us both, but in the main, this agreement worked well.

So, for much of our married life, Ralph and I had a small circle of individuals whose friendship with us was no older than our marriage. As a result, in essence Ralph had spent most of our married life in a solitary way, waiting for me to come home from work, as he retired within six or seven years of our marriage owing to his failing physical health. The exception to that were his children, who had continued to be a central part of our shared lives. Despite his failing health, when we were able to, we joined in birthdays and family celebrations with the growing grandchildren and their parents. That continued to bring Ralph and me so much happiness.

Ralph had never been what I would class a 'joiner', in that he never joined or was an active member or part of any organisation or body apart from the church. When I was working and he was at home all day, I had so often encouraged him to try to get involved in something, but he just wasn't interested. Over the years, I had to come to accept that that was just the way he was, and what he was comfortable with. When physically able, Ralph had played an active role in our local church, but as the years had passed, so his church life had become passive and receptive as opposed to active and giving, before teetering out altogether. Neither was he an avid reader or an ardent hobbyist, or a collector of bizarre objects or memorabilia. As a consequence of all of this, he had led a very quiet, self-contained life for the years before I retired, and so when I was permanently around the home, it provided much-wanted company and stimulation for him. It also had the added bonus, as I believe he saw it, of letting him finally cede personal and household control to me.

At the start of this new year, it was as if the early days of my retirement were being repeated, as after the special Christmas we'd had, once again I had the impression that he just let go and slumped into himself physically and mentally. Ralph seemed to once again relinquish what little there was left of his remaining will to contribute to being involved in his own life or lifestyle. In retrospect, I realised that perhaps he had drawn on whatever inner resilience and strength he had to give us that wonderful shared Christmas, and I was amazed that he had been able to foresee and plan to do that, let alone achieve it. However, as we began this new year together, it became apparent that what had been a wonderful Christmas time between us had been just that: a unique limited period of time, which now sadly was over.

It seemed to me, as the month of January moved on, that our lives were just disintegrating into a further separation of the conjoined and mutual lives that we both loved. What was so much worse for me was that I could do absolutely nothing but watch it go.

The new year brought unfamiliar snow, sleet and ice along with bitterly cold and strong winds that meant we were not able to get out as much as we had been doing. The icy roads and pavements were challenging enough for me to contend with, let alone Ralph. We stayed indoors and enjoyed the comfort and warmth of our home with log fires, watching television together when we could and enjoying the peacefulness of lying on the top of the bed for hours on end. However, this month signalled the start of Ralph not asking to go out, and when I suggested it, he often said, 'You go. I'll stay here.' When we did get out, we were now down to only two or three coffee shops that were suitable for us in that they were near home, required only minimal walking on his part, or were very easily managed with a wheelchair. I was also increasingly unhappy to leave him sitting in the car while I scurried around our local town and did some shopping, so I tried to coordinate my shopping and appointments to coincide with my afternoons off, or when his daughters sat with him to enable me to go out.

Ralph had, by early in this new January, reverted to his familiar pattern of sleeping for hours each day. As the month continued, Ralph's life seemed to consist of him lying, sleeping and going out only when I encouraged, if not forced, him to do so. I was so determined to keep him up and about that I continued to encourage him to walk as much as I felt was possible for him to do safely, to get outdoors if only for a drive in the car, and to take any opportunities we could to engage with family both in and, importantly, outside the home. However, he was not a willing participant in these activities and inevitably, when I was strapping him into the car, he would often ask, 'How long will we be here?' or, 'When will we be home?'

So, after the joy that was Christmas, the first few weeks of the new year brought back to me, with razor-like clarity, the reality of the relentlessness of the continued decline that was our 'D' journey. New and unexpected changes and challenges seemed to come one after another for us both. In particular, the zoned-out periods became even more frequent and lasted for about a day and a half. It was frightening to watch Ralph during these times. He stared into space with his eyes and mouth wide open. He could not respond to any instructions, and when he was like this I had no option but to leave him in his pyjamas and keep him in the bedroom. I got into the habit of checking him every fifteen minutes when I had left him lying sleeping and was doing some household chore in the kitchen. I found myself from time to time standing at the bedroom door waiting to see his chest move to assure myself that he was still breathing, so ghastly did he look at times.

He had no idea who I was, where he was and what was happening in or to his body during these times. He lost all control of bodily functions and movements, becoming incontinent and unable to feed himself or hold a cup to take a drink. It seemed as if we had just got over one zoned-out period when I could see in him the tell-tale signs that another one was on its way. It was exhausting for both him and me, and during these days we both just slept and ate when I could get him settled enough to do either. When these times passed it took me a day to regain my own strength, get all the necessary washing up to date, and encourage Ralph to eat and drink to make up for what he had lost in the days before.

This new phase of physical and mental deterioration brought me to the realisation that our days of being able to muddle together alone were coming to an end, and that, reluctantly but necessarily, it was time to seek more help. I struggled on as long as I could, but by the time we were into the double dates of the month, I had to admit defeat and request more help with his personal care. I discussed the need to do this with Ralph on one of his more rational days and he appeared to understand what I was saying, but what made it even more difficult and sad for me was that it didn't seem to bother him at all. Ralph's acceptance of the need to allow others to help with his personal care was unnerving, and his willingness to allow others to work with him at these most personal of times really upset me. As always at these times, when able, he just said, 'Whatever you think best, dear.'

My forgotten birthday

My birthday comes around early in the year, and over the previous twenty-seven years that Ralph and I had been together, we had always marked it by doing something special. This twenty-eighth time was different. Ralph forgot it, or, to be more accurate, by now he could not differentiate one day from another, and so when reminded on the February morning that it was my birthday, he just did not see any relevance in that fact for him. In 2017, the birthday just before Ralph received his diagnosis, I had reminded him that it was my birthday, and when we were out for a coffee a few days before it, I had helped him buy a card for me. He had even managed to write his name and put a few kisses on the card himself, which meant so much at the time and meant even more as I reflected on it this year.

The previous year had been a special birthday and so I had encouraged him to 'take me out' for lunch. I thought that by that stage in his condition, as we awaited the appointment that would give us the diagnosis I knew was coming, that lunch would be a lot easier than going out for an evening meal, something we hadn't done in years. We went to a favourite restaurant and had a very pleasant lunch in some regards, but it was evident that it was all a bit much for him, and in reality for me too. Ralph couldn't read the menu, and when the meal I picked for him came, he just looked at it and couldn't work out how to eat it. I had chosen a pastry pie for him. In honour of the occasion, I had overcome my reluctance to give Ralph pies, and on this special day for us both I thought that he should have something he really liked to help him remember it. When his food came it was an individual dish of pie filling with a separately cooked and then set on top pastry crouton, which I was singularly unimpressed with. Ralph just looked at it. I ended up having to upend the dish and scoop the pie filling out onto his plate. He just looked at this unfamiliar food and needed my direction and encouragement to pick up his cutlery and eat his meal. He was visibly uncomfortable, if not frightened, sitting in the middle of this unfamiliar place with lots of noisy, strange people, and so as soon as we had eaten our main course, I got us both a coffee and the bill. That was our last meal out together.

This year when I reminded Ralph on the morning that it was my birthday, he asked, 'Is it, indeed?' and then, in a very formal fashion, wished me a happy birthday. I asked him if he would like to get a card for me. He thought for a minute and said, 'Yes, you buy a card for yourself, dear,' so I did. I bought a card and set it in front of him later and asked him if he could write his name on it for me. I gave him the pen and he put it to the card and then drew a lovely curved line over the place in the card where you would normally write. I told him that was lovely, but could he try to write his name on the card. Ralph put pen to card again, and to my surprise managed to write a fairly legible signature. When he had finished this laborious task, he looked up at me and smiled. I laughed with him and asked him if he was going to give me a few kisses on the card, and he bent down to the task again and carefully marked two wobbly x's underneath his name. I treasure it.

Later that evening he remarked on the cards on the coffee table and asked what they were. I reminded him that it was my birthday and showed him the card he had written for me. He said he hoped that I would have a very happy birthday and could he go to bed.

Sharing Ralph's caring

As I lay on the bed beside Ralph that birthday night, I thought about control. I have, I am ashamed to admit, always been a controlling type of person. I like to lead, not follow, make and take decisions, and am not in the least spontaneous, preferring to have a clear plan, not just go with the flow. I like to write lists and tick them off, to be clear about when and where things are done and, if at all possible, to have a daily and weekly routine to follow. Over the previous years this skill had come into its own as Ralph was only too keen to let me organise and plan our lives, for me to lead and him to follow. Ralph's release of control had been balanced by my taking more control and, if I was honest, that suited me just fine. However, as I thought about the control I now wielded on his and our lives, I realised that the time had come for me – just as he had done at the time of my retirement, and indeed prior to it – to cede that control to others. The rapid decline in Ralph's health that I saw in this new year meant that if I continued to exert and control his life by myself, I would not be serving his best interests. I needed to accept that there were professionals who could and should now assess and respond to his changing physical and mental health needs, and whom I should now support in that, rather than me control who should support him and us both.

I thought about John the Baptist and those famous words he said: 'He [Jesus] must become greater; I must become less' (John 3:30). All my life I had driven myself to be the best, to be in the front and lead, to be known and acknowledged for the work that I did, and I had enjoyed a career that allowed me to achieve those things in a limited but real way. I had relished it.

Even as I set off on my caring journey, I was happy to be the contact person; to take the phone calls, to sit opposite the health and social care professionals and

131

provide them with information on which decisions about Ralph's future would be jointly made, then for me to carry out those decisions myself from a position of control. But now the reality hit me with force that I was getting to a place that was outside my ability to make and control those decisions. Ralph's needs had become greater than I could cope with by myself, and were taking him and me into grey and dark areas that were and would be strange to us both. The time had come for the professionals to be in control, to tell me what needed to be done and to advise or instruct me in how to do it. I didn't like that but I had to accept it, not begrudgingly but graciously. I had to become less directly involved in his care and let others take a more dominant role. That would not be easy, but it was necessary.

Courteousness

Many years ago, Ralph and I attended a Sunday evening meeting in a local Gospel Hall where a very gracious senior saintly man gave a lovely word on courteousness, based on the verse, 'Finally, be ye all of one mind, having compassion one of another, love as brethren, be pitiful, be courteous' (1 Peter 3:8, AKJV).

He talked about how in today's world so many people are discourteous in their dealings with people, and sadly he had noted that trait in some Christians. He strongly advised us as Christians to be courteous in our dealings with others, particularly with those of no or other faiths, so that they could see the love of Christ in us in how we interacted with them.

I had to accept that sometimes in my efforts to be in control throughout my life I had been less than courteous with those I had interacted with. To my deep regret, there were times in the past when I had been too often clinical in my determination to ensure, if at all possible, that my preferred way forward was followed when others, including Ralph, had different viewpoints. Acknowledging this, I knew that I did not want to repeat this approach in my attitude to other people who now needed to both direct and share in his care needs.

Having come to the point where I accepted that I needed to give up my total control over Ralph's 'D' life and seek and follow others' guidance on what would be best for him, I knew that I needed to do this courteously and humbly. I knew that I would not find this easy, but not doing it was not an option, as new people would have to come into his and my life and we would all have to build and nurture mutual relationships with each other.

I can still see that saint, standing up in that meeting and smiling as he quietly encouraged his listeners in that country Gospel Hall to be courteous, to be Christlike and, above all, to be Christian.[11]

As the month drew to an end and I waited for the professionals to come to assess Ralph's current needs and advise on what help was now required, I prayed that I would be courteous in my interactions, that I would graciously cede my control, accept their advice and support and be humble in my dealings with them. In short, that I would be Christlike.

---

[11] As remembered from an evening message on this passage, given in a Gospel Hall, Northern Ireland, circa 1996.

11
Think Positively

There is only so much negativity than anyone can cope with at any one time. A small amount in the tapestry of our lives provides shade and nuance and helps us appreciate the good things that come along to balance it. However, too much weighs us down as we try to cope with the difficulties or challenges we are going through. It is one of the peculiarities of life that difficult times are so often made worse by other small, insignificant, negative events that under normal circumstances we would sail through without a thought, but when experienced in conjunction with daily or unexpected problems in our lives, they assume monumental proportions.

Why is it that when we are feeling down, or a bit depressed or weary with the repetitive routine and challenges of life, it always seems that the washing machine breaks or we fall and twist an ankle or get toothache, or lose a favourite earring or glove? Add such minor upsets to what we have to deal with at difficult times and their cumulative effects can cause us to lose control or snap. The final straw can be when the person or people we look to for support or encouragement at these times are on holiday, or have a cold, or are totally absorbed with their own family and therefore are not available for us.

Focus on the important

Very early in our married life, Ralph and I took a fairly mundane but, over time, what proved to be an extremely significant decision. We decided not to watch any soap operas on television. In the first couple of years together, we had got into the habit of having our tea in front of the TV while we watched nightly episodes of a number of soap operas. One storyline had me particularly intrigued and I remember cancelling meeting up with someone so that I could watch a particular episode. These were the days before on-demand options were available. Some days later, Ralph asked me why I hadn't gone to meet that individual. When I told him, he just looked at me, obviously disappointed, and asked me how I could prioritise characters in a soap opera over a real friend. When he put it like that, I have to admit that I was ashamed.

As we talked about it, we agreed that we would be better occupied eating our dinner at the kitchen table and spending that time talking to each other about our real lives and the people we had met that day, not watching make-believe characters and their dysfunctional lives on TV. We kept to that decision, and while, of course, we continued to watch and enjoy certain television programmes, we were careful about not getting too embroiled in dramas or serials to the detriment of us being fully engaged in our lives in the real world.

Ralph's progressively deteriorating health really started to upset me. I kept looking at him, seeing him failed and failing, sleeping so much, zoned out so much. I was tired and weary. It was cold and icy. I'd had one household bill after another. The garage door broke. I had windows that didn't shut properly and there seemed to me to be a force nine gale coming through them. The back gate wouldn't open or shut properly. A new iron I had bought only months before was spitting dirty water out at me, and my favourite pair of earrings broke. There were weeks when I was having to do washing two if not several times every day because of all the clean sheets and clothes I needed to have on hand. To cap it all, every time I turned on the television at night after Ralph was tucked up in bed, hoping for some light relief, all I could find to watch were endless repeats. I didn't even want to use my on-demand option, as I was so tired. I only wanted something that lasted about thirty minutes, as that was all the length of time that I had the energy to concentrate on. The news was totally depressing. It was all too much.

As Ralph continued to visibly decline in front of me and as I was seemingly surrounded by this cloud of negativity all around me, once again I found myself feeling that heavy burden on my shoulders, wearing me down and wearying me. No matter how much sleep I got, I woke each morning feeling exhausted. My nights were now usually disturbed two or three times, as Ralph needed to get up to go to the toilet, or during his zoned-out times when he was unable to do this, I needed to get him up to change him. It all seemed too much, and I could feel myself getting a bit down and even sad, to the point of feeling sorry for myself. I tried to pull myself out of it, but it was hard, and as I waited to see what extra help I would need and receive, the unending physical toll of it all seemed too much to bear. When I tried to look up and around me, all I could see in the news or on the television totally depressed me. When I was out and about, I found myself getting angry at other drivers who I thought were rude and aggressive. I felt that assistants in shops and offices were dismissive of me, and I couldn't believe the litter that people threw out of their cars onto the sides of the road, or the carpet of chewing gum on pavements. Had people no shame?!

I decided at this time that I couldn't take all the negativity that seemed to be piling up in my life and pulling me down. I couldn't change the way Ralph's health was deteriorating, but I could change some other things to help me cope better with those. I started writing lists and worked my way through them, first tackling those practical issues that were really annoying me. I got the garage door fixed, then the windows, then I bought a new iron. I bought new bed linen so that I could wash full loads at a time, and bought extra changes of clothes for Ralph. Remembering the decision that we had made together all those years ago, I decided that I would not watch the news on television any more. I couldn't cope with all the shootings and wars and evil and power lust that seemed to make up so much of it. It just depressed me too much, so I turned the radio on and listened instead to classical music, which calmed me. I needed more positivity in my life, so I bought special teas to drink in the afternoons when Ralph slept, and treated myself to some new everyday clothes so that I was at least clean and tidy and felt better about myself around the house.

Unexpected kindnesses

As I sat and drank my nice tea, I found myself thinking of the many blessings I had received during this and previous, similar times when life had seemed beyond bearable and I wanted out, or at least I wanted out for the duration of the difficulties I was facing. I remembered those unexpected acts of kindness that had come along when I most needed them but didn't expect them and so often didn't even realise that they were such acts until after the event.

The man who came to fix my windows noticed that my back gate didn't shut properly, so without asking, and because he had a drill in his hand, he took off the bolt and repositioned it so that it opened and closed securely. The couple who came to visit us from our church sent out a catalogue they had used for aids and adaptations which proved so useful to me for Ralph's needs. All my neighbours checked with me during the bad weather when we were housebound for a couple of days to see if there was anything we needed that they could get for us. Lynda turned up one day with some soup she had made for us, and Gwen arrived with lovely bunches of colourful spring flowers to cheer both me and the house up, and a sweet treat to enjoy with a coffee. My sister, Liz, sent me a book she had read and been encouraged by in her own Christian journey and which heartened me. Some friends from my former workplace met up with me for lunch – Wilma came and sat with her dad to let me go out to meet them.

I was so blessed, if only I would take the time to look up from feeling sorry for myself and see it.

I thought about the boy in the Bible story who went along to hear Jesus (John 6:1-13). He had brought his packed lunch and when he realised that everyone else around him was hungry and that the people who were with the preacher were frantically looking for food to feed them, he stood up in the middle of that melee and gave the disciples his few pieces of bread and cold fish for them to share. I remembered the little Israeli girl who was taken from her home and trafficked, to use a modern word, to become a servant in the home of an army commander in Syria. She shared with her mistress what she knew about a prophet who could heal the commander of his leprosy, and because of her intervention, Naaman was wonderfully healed (2 Kings 5).

What both of these unnamed, seemingly insignificant, anonymous young people had in common was that they cared about others. The boy was not selfish, or self-centred, and the girl did not feel sorry for herself because of the situation she was in through no fault of her own. They didn't hold back what they had for themselves when they saw the needs of others. Instead, they freely gave what seemingly little or insignificant resource they had to benefit those around them. The amazing part of these stories for me is that if these two young people had held on to what they had – their lunch and their information – the likelihood was that no one would have been any the wiser. No one would have noticed that boy among the 5,000 men on the hillside that day if he hadn't stood up and spoken up and given up his lunch. No one would ever have asked that little servant girl if she knew anyone who could heal her master, given the status of women and servants in the society she found herself living in.

As I reflected on the kindnesses of others to me, I felt like one of those 5,000 (and more) people in the crowd who suddenly received an unexpected gift of food at a time when I was so very needy, or, like Naaman, thrown a lifeline, even if I didn't appreciate it at the time. Those recent unexpected acts of kindness, and so many more kindnesses I came to realise I had been the recipient of over the previous months, nourished and encouraged me, strengthened me for the onward journey and gave me hope. There was so much good around, if I could only lift my eyes up from the cares and negativity that were pulling me down.

I remembered two pieces I had written months before when I was in a similar state of mind. I had obviously seen some news on the television that saddened and depressed me, and this moved me to scribble down some thoughts on what I felt about it. Perhaps it is an Ulster idiom to say that you are 'pushed' when the pressures of life get too much, but it does express in a very straightforward way how you can feel when things overwhelm you. Sometimes it can feel as if everything around you is just pushing you out of control and towards breaking point and there is nothing you can do about it.

As I reflected on what I had written about being pushed, and then seeing others in other countries or in other situations who were being pushed far beyond what I could ever cope with, I realised that there is the other side of that experience. Where there is action there is always a counter action. Where there is pushing in the sense that I experienced it in my life, or saw others experience it in theirs, there was also the counter movement of goodness, of kindness, of help and of support. How amazing it is that unexpected gifts so very often come when they are least expected, at the most challenging and difficult times we face, and can be given by those from whom they would never be expected.

People Are Pushed

People are pushed
Beyond what they can bear and towards what is
    unknown
The world too small for all the hate and pain
    therein
Individuals too insignificant to be counted
    individually
The thousands, the ethnics, the castes and
    classes
Moving like locusts, carried by the winds of
    change
Blown to closed doors and barbed wire and
    uniformed controllers
To tented ghettos and bottled water and
    unfamiliar food
No home, no work, no pride, dependent on
    charity reluctantly given
Wanting so much and wanted so little.

People are pushed
Along with the herd and into the pens of
    fashion and stuff
Where there is never enough, always more
    wanted and then some
Where toil and graft and heft and repetition of
    effort
Build up frustration and envy of others unseen
    and unknown
Blame apportioned liberally but away from self
Offence taken so readily and given so freely
Words pushed out into the ether without
    thinking of consequences
Rights push back courtesy and our wants
    supersede others' needs
It's all about me, not you; us, not them.

People are pushed
In their heads and hearts to places they don't
    know or recognise
To think thoughts and say words they never
    should
To join others in actions of hate they never
    thought they would or could
To where acts of kindness are so random, they
    are ridiculed as weakness
The herded become the herders, the persecuted
    the persecutors
And charity is a dirty word spat out, curled up,
    trampled upon and rare
Pain inflicted for pleasure, but for the receiver,
    only pain

Disclosure buried under layers of subterfuge
    and protected by law
Anonymity flaunted by all and privacy
    protected by so few
It's our lives, our country, our world.

I don't like it.

People Are Moved

People are moved
By forces within and without to do unexpected
    deeds
To achieve things they and others believed they
    never could
The silent, the ordinary, the unnoticed masses
    have been moved
To write words that stir hearts and say words
    that cause others to right wrongs
To march on work days and have car stickers
    that support the cause
To stand up for and with the dishonoured and
    those with no voice
To shed tears for all the inhumanities suffered
    by the many
And feel shame for the ease of life afforded to
    the few.

People are moved
To leave home and hearth and all things
    familiar
To go to places unknown and countries hard to
    spell

To pack rucksacks and buy new boots and get
    injections for the arriving
To live in the same tents and eat the same grain
    as those they seek to help
Working in mud and poor light and with
    children with runny noses
Prepared to offer presence and kindness,
    laughter and a wash
To hold a grandfather's hand and cry with a
    despairing mother
To listen not talk, sit not stand, and share a lice-
    infested bed.

People are moved
From all countries and places, not just ours or
    theirs
From all castes and classes and genders or none
The excluded and vulnerable, the affected and
    disaffected
Led to others, for others and with others to do
    the old-fashioned thing
To give and not to count the cost, to serve
    without seeking reward[12]
Why? Because their hearts are too full and their
    hands always open
To even the odds, reduce the gap, equal the
    inequalities and draw a line in the sand
Over which there is no movement.

I like Movers.

---

[12] Adapted from the 'Prayer of Ignatius of Loyola',
www.prayerfoundation.org/prayer_of_ignatius_of_loyola.htm
(accessed 11th December 2020).

When faced with the challenges of life, we each have a choice how to respond to them. We can be pushed or counter move. We can sit down or stand up. We can speak up or stay quiet. We can give or wait to receive. We can be instigators of pain or individuals who help or support. We can demonstrate positivity or negativity in our attitude and demeanour during these experiences. The choice is ours.

Sometimes, however, our choices are limited to the point of being non-existent, and if and when this is the case, we have to hope that other people can help and support us in difficult times, by the choices and subsequent actions they take, however seemingly small or insignificant those choices may appear to be to them. Like the boy in the story of the feeding of the 5,000 or the little servant girl in the healing of Naaman, or those individuals who helped me during this challenging time, small actions by others can have huge and lasting positive consequences for us as individuals and within our communities and our society.

Ralph and I both had great cause to thank God for people in our lives who chose to move close to us at this time. The practical help and support they gave to us was humbling, perhaps even more so because they most likely didn't realise the impact that it had on our lives. To see and then be moved to help those who need support at a particular time in their lives is a wonderful gift and, I believe, God-inspired. We were so blessed that others around us at these challenging and difficult times on our 'D' journey used their choices to help, surprise, support and care for us. I'm sure these individuals may never fully appreciate how much they did for us, or how much it meant to us, but the choices they made then would be remembered not just by me, and I hoped by Ralph, but surely also by God.

Like the widow Jesus noticed in the temple (Luke 21:1-4), it is not how much you have, but how much of what you have that you share with others that is your legacy.

12
At Home

Having accepted, at the end of January, that I needed to ask for more assistance with Ralph's care, a number of assessments of his personal care needs were carried out by the appropriate health and social care professionals in early February. Shortly afterwards, much-appreciated support arrived in the form of a range of practical aids to help with his incontinence. I had to clear out a wardrobe to house all the products I was now being supplied with to address his continence needs. However, that minor inconvenience of less space for clothes was more than compensated for with the reduction in the amount of washing and tumble drying I needed to do, and by the security and comfort he got from the aids. To my surprise and delight, Ralph accepted the need to wear the pads in his clothing really well and didn't mind them. What a relief, in one way. How sad in another.

After the most recent really bad zoned-out time, which seemed to last for days and was particularly draining for us both, but especially for Ralph, I kept waiting for the next bad time to come. I waited and waited but it did not come as I expected. What had arrived in its place, or perhaps, to be more accurate, what was left of Ralph after the last zoned-out time he had gone through, was nearly worse. It took me a couple of weeks to realise that since that last bad time, his recovery had not been as good as it had been in times past, and that the man now with me had significantly deteriorated from what he had been even a few weeks before. Unlike those previous times, Ralph did not regain his renewed energy or interest in life and living. Sadly, it became evident that he seemed to have moved down another gear in his ability to engage with or participate in life.

Ralph now never wanted to get out of bed, nor did he want to go out anywhere. He wouldn't sit up on the couch and watch television, preferring to watch it from a lying-down position in bed. He was totally disinterested in his food, now always needing to be coaxed and encouraged to eat and drink. His shoulders were slumped; he was so stooped over. He winced and gasped sometimes when he was moving or getting up from a lying position, and I realised he must be in pain from his arthritis and bad back. He was just failing in every aspect of his life, physically, mentally and emotionally. It was sad and distressing to watch. When people called in to see him, he smiled as usual, and when they asked him how he was he always said he was good, or he would laugh and say, 'Not bad.' But he had absolutely no idea who he was talking to or what their relationship to him was, and when they had gone, he had no recollection of them being there or that he had spent time with them. He was quiet to the point of withdrawn, and would just sit, when I could persuade him to do that, or lie on the bed, staring ahead of him for what seemed like hours on end.

Home became a big issue again in that Ralph now never thought he was at home. This was the start of him asking me repeatedly every day if he could go home. Worryingly for me, he always looked so sad when he asked that question. I realised that he never recognised where he was now as his home. Home was not here. Where exactly it was and whether it was the same home that he wanted to go to each time he asked me to take him there was also not clear. Frequently when he had been changed into his pyjamas and was lying in bed at night, he would look up at me and with huge, fearful eyes ask, 'Why will you not take me home?'

Often, he first asked me if I had a car, then where it was and if I could drive it. When he had got those issues clear in his mind, he would plead with me to take him home. I asked him time and time again where home was, who was there, what it looked like, but he rarely answered. Only once did he come up with a previous house, one he had lived in almost fifty years earlier – long before we were together. When I asked who lived in this house with him, he couldn't tell me, he just said he wanted to go there.

During these times Ralph was obviously distressed and upset that he wasn't at home as he understood that term. It broke my heart that he was not content where he was and not content with me, and so desperately wanted to be somewhere else. I said that home for me was where he was, and that home for him was where I was, and that home was where we lived together now. He usually accepted this explanation at the time, and when I asked him if he was happy to be with me now in this home, he said he was, but it didn't stop the question being asked several times each day. It was as if every day when Ralph woke up either in the morning or after a sleep in the middle of the day, he felt like it was a whole new place he woke up in. An unfamiliar one, a scary one and one he wanted to leave.

Unsettling times

During our married life we had been serial house movers. It became something of a family joke, even a family myth, how many times we moved. We just seemed to up sticks every few years, or in one case after only ten months, to live in a new house. Mostly it was Ralph's idea. I remember coming home from work one day and he said to me that 'we' were selling the house and moving to a new development less than a mile away. I asked him who 'we' were since I thought 'we' meant him and me, but as he hadn't discussed this fairly significant decision with me, who was the other half of the 'we' he was talking about? Without even a smile at my attempt at a joke, he simply said it was the estate agent, and they had both agreed it was time for us to move. So we moved, and less than four years later we moved again. I knew from what his family had told me that frequent house moves had also been a feature of their life as children.

I wonder about that now – Ralph being unsettled in any house he lived in after spending some time there, and needing to move to find somewhere new and different. Something somewhere in his DNA or formative years meant he couldn't rest for long periods of time in one place. In that trait, we were very alike. I too had been a serial mover in the early part of my life, though my moving genre was countries, not houses. I chose to leave Northern Ireland to go to college in Scotland and then I chose to go away to Papua New Guinea for two years as a volunteer. When I returned from that, I did begin to work at home but couldn't really settle, and within two years had decided to leave again and headed off to Nepal for three years.

It was after returning from there that I met Ralph, and when we were getting to know each other and beginning to realise that we might want to consider marriage, he asked me outright if I wanted or needed to go away again. I was always very clear from when I accepted his marriage proposal that my life was with him, and wherever he wanted to be, I would be right there beside him. But despite my assurances, as our relationship developed there remained times when I realised that Ralph did worry that I might want or need to go abroad again. On one occasion, shortly before we were married, he shared with me that he thought if anything were to happen to him, I would most likely go away again. I never thought that, but no matter how much I tried to reassure him about this, for whatever reason he was never totally convinced. I believe the thought that I would want to go abroad again troubled him many times during our marriage.

That temporary dwelling concept in relation to all the houses we lived in came to an end with our current home. In all our previous houses, Ralph and I had decorated or redecorated them in what the hosts of property shows on television would call 'neutral' colours. Soft whites, beiges and even the dreaded magnolia were the palettes of our choice. We were also both minimalist in our approach to décor and possessions. Neither of us collected anything, most likely an obvious consequence of our previous frequent moving lifestyles, and so our houses were simply, though I hope tastefully, decorated and definitely uncluttered. Easy dusting from my perspective, less to pack up from Ralph's. I only realised how temporarily we regarded all of our previous houses when our estate agent, by now nearly a personal friend, was in our neighbourhood meeting a client and popped in to see us about two years after he had completed the sale on the house we were living in at that time. After a cup of tea, he asked if he could take a walk around the house to see what we had done with it. When he came back to the lounge after doing this, he was smiling and shaking his head and said that he would happily take any prospective buyer around our house that minute as it was in showing condition. That was when I realised that I always kept the house we were in as a *house*. I didn't allow them to ever become a *home*. We always decorated and maintained our houses with a view to moving on.

The longest we had ever stayed in any one house prior to where we now live was four years, and it took our current home to buck that trend. While it was not a self-build, we did get significant input into the interior room layout and size. As by that stage Ralph's mobility problems were becoming very evident, we took the opportunity with this house to plan it to accommodate his increasing mobility and physical needs. We tried as best we could to future-proof its layout and facilities for what might come along later for him. I knew that we were likely to stay here for the duration of our lives when, four years after we bought it, we redecorated two rooms and put coloured paint on the walls. That was the first really bright paint we had used in a house in twenty years. I knew then we had found our forever home on earth.

Our heavenly home

Both of us grew up going to many gospel meetings during our childhood and adolescence. These evangelical outreach meetings were held in small country churches, halls or even in draughty tents and were held nightly for two weeks or depending on the attendance, perhaps even for a month. They were conducted by self-styled, often self-taught itinerant lay preachers or evangelists who, regardless of what they lacked in theological accuracy or biblical training, more than compensated for in the drama and forcefulness of their nightly delivery. They were salesmen, experts in communication, and often direct to the point of accusative in their message. Nightly they harangued pews full of willing listeners, and not a few individuals cajoled into being there by parents or neighbours.

Some of my earliest memories are of being crammed into pews or sitting on uncomfortable, foldable metal chairs in my Sunday-best outfit and holding my head down while the preacher bellowed, gesticulated and thumped the pulpit for what seemed like hours, hearing the 'Amens' and 'Praise the Lords' rebound around the meeting when a particularly popular point was made. Most frequently, the word of the night was 'hell'. These preachers had an unshakable belief and deeply held concern about the possible damnation of the unsaved souls in front of them. They believed with certainty in the second coming of our Saviour and had a very real fear that not everyone in the gathering before them would be saved before the time of the rapture,[13] which they believed to be imminent. It led them to pour their hearts and souls into trying to lead their listeners to salvation. Their preaching made for uncomfortable listening for children, let alone some of the adults who attended, and there was many a night I wondered if we would make it home before Jesus would come again.

Those hellfire preachers of yesteryear might come in for criticism today, but no one could doubt their burden for unsaved souls and their desire to use every breath they had to preach the gospel. Perhaps today, while some might not wish to go back to those times, we might do well to recognise our sanitisation of sin in our lives and acknowledge our acquiescence to the secular standards of the materialistic world we live in. We also need to admit our tendency today to stay quiet on the challenges of the eternal certainties as we understand them to be taught in the Bible.

Central to the hell message these preachers thundered out nightly was the alternative certainty of heaven and, contrary to its damnable opposing destination, it was always spoken of either softly with tenderness or loudly

---

[13] When Jesus is believed to snatch His Church away. See 1 Thessalonians 4:16-18.

with triumph and celebration. A place to be desired and gained. A place of happiness, contentment, perpetual worship and often compared with home. Our heavenly home; our home in the sky; our eternal home; our home beyond and our final home. A home from which once entered there would be no leaving, no feeling of being unsettled or of being there as a temporary resident. It was a forever home, a final place of resting, a home for the soul.

As I recalled these vivid memories of forceful end-time preaching from my childhood, I reflected on where Ralph and I were on our eternal journey. Our 'D' journey was meandering along, taking twists and turns as it did so, and we were going with its flow, with God's help. Like all Christians, we had both been taught and believed that our Christian journey would ultimately lead us to heaven, at a time and in a manner of God's choosing. And, as with most Christians, while we believed that and had assurance that it would come one day, we did not dwell on it obsessively or fear the means by which we would realise our heavenly reward. Rather, the assurance of it was like a warm blanket that we always kept in a cupboard. We knew it was there, but we only took it out when we needed its warmth and security at times of cold or bitter experiences.

Home for Ralph and me now was both temporal and temporary. After a life of wandering as unsettled house owners, we had found our earthly home in our present house. Home, as the world understands the use of that term, is often thought of as being where our heart finds rest and contentment. It is a place where those we love and feel safe with are. To me, this was exactly what our current house was and would always be, and so I was saddened that it was not always a recognisable safe and heartfelt home to Ralph at this time. I continued to assure him that he was home. Home with me and home to stay.

However, I also had a renewed sense at this time that our journey would ultimately lead us, like it leads all of saved humanity, to our eternal home. A home where Ralph and I would be heavenly residents, would feel completely at home and would never want to leave. I did not need to focus on when we might eventually arrive at our eternal home, or what would be the means or cause by which we would reach it. Rather, having the assurance that reaching it was God's promise to us was a great comfort as I focused on the daily challenges and pleasures of our lives here on earth.

Our earthly home was the safe haven that provided a refuge from all the buffeting and challenges we experienced on our 'D' journey and a constant in all the changes we faced along the way. I felt totally at peace in it, and while Ralph did not, I feared that perhaps with his deteriorating memory he would never feel completely at ease in it ever again. Nevertheless, I took comfort in the fact that one day he would be at home; an eternal home that he would recognise all the time, feel settled and happy in and never want to leave. I hoped and prayed that God would spare us to enjoy our earthly home together for many more years, but whenever his or my time here on earth was over, I knew that one day Ralph and I would be united again in our heavenly home for ever and that would be 'far better' (Philippians 1:23, AKJV).

13

One Year's Journey Completed

We had made it. One year had passed from when Ralph and I sat in that health centre and got his 'D' diagnosis, and we were still here. In one way, it all seemed so long ago, as if things had always been this way, and yet in the extraordinary contradiction that is time, it seemed like only yesterday since we were both trying to take in the enormity of it, attempting to make some sense of it all. Yet here we were, one year later. Together. Different yet the same, the same yet different, changed yet the essence of us both unchanged and only too well aware that change and difference would be our future.

Just like the new year that had come and gone, we didn't mark the event. It was just another day in our home, with the same routine and the same challenges to be overcome, but as I reflected on the milestone that the day heralded, I did realise the significance of it for us both. When we had officially set out on this 'D' journey one year earlier, we really had no idea where we would end up one month ahead, let alone one year later. In that we were no different from anyone else, because who of us knows what a day, let alone a month or year, will bring. But for Ralph and me, we accepted that the added burden of Ralph's diagnosis was likely to bring us more than our expected share of unknowns. One year on and we had now replaced some of those unknowns with known, but many more unknowns remained. As I allowed myself the luxury of looking back on this significant day, I thought about both of those opposing categories.

One year on, what did I know? Well, I knew Ralph certainly was physically and mentally frailer than he had been one year before, but I was not at all sure which state had deteriorated more or which had contributed more to the overall erosion of his health. Physically he was alarmingly doddery, less sure on his feet, more prone to losing his balance and as such needed more support. He now automatically used his rollator around the home rather than the walking stick he had used a year previously, and he could never walk anywhere outside the home without someone holding on to him. He also now needed help getting out of a chair or the car seat, and both inside and outside the home he needed guidance as to where he was going, as he had no idea where the kitchen was in relation to his bedroom or which was our car in a car park. He now couldn't put his shoes or slippers on and couldn't do up buttons on his shirt, or put a jumper or cardigan on. In terms of his mental health, he was more often than not unresponsive in word and scarily vacant in his eye and facial expressions. He never initiated a conversation and seldom responded directly to one being conducted with him. He looked and listened, but rarely gave any indication that he was following what was being said or was aware of what was going on. Ralph was passive and placid, weak and weary, quiet and eerily calm.

What did I not know? I did not know what Ralph was thinking or feeling, and that upset me as he couldn't always tell me, which meant that I would never really know if or when he was sad, unhappy or anxious. He couldn't tell me or show me, apart from the rare word or expression at a particularly difficult or happy event, that he was feeling any emotion at all, and that reality kept me awake some nights. I so wanted him to have at least some happiness and joy in his life, but it was hard to know most of the time if that was possible, let alone if he might be experiencing it. I didn't know if the pace of Ralph's decline was normal for someone with his diagnosis, exceptional in either speed or delay, or unusual in any medical or psychological way, and no one could tell me if it was, as of course everyone experiences dementia in their own unique way. I did not know if the medication Ralph was on was helping him, doing him no harm or impairing his condition. I did not know what tomorrow would be like and so couldn't plan or commit to anything beyond a day ahead. When planning any event with others, I was always having to put in the caveat that yes, we could do that or go there provided he was OK on the day.

Lost...

During my career I worked for more than twenty years for the same health and social care organisation, having a variety of roles and positions that moved me around and through its hierarchical structures. About ten years after I began working with it, the entire workforce moved premises. It was a mammoth achievement to move a number of departments, their staff and office equipment, not to mention their resources, which at the time ran to tons of paper records and files. So, to facilitate this, a schedule of moving specific departments and their staff to the new premises was developed. This was drawn up to minimise disruption for the work of the organisation itself, and, more importantly, to enable other external agencies and clients who interacted with it to continue to do so on a daily basis throughout the entire moving process.

The department I was working in at the time was scheduled to move over a weekend, which meant that we were to have packed up by a Friday afternoon and the moving firm would then have our office furniture, boxes and files in our new offices for us when we arrived at the new site on the following Monday morning. Needless to say, while we were all happy for the moving firm to take the majority of our stuff to the new building, there were personal bits and pieces that we had in our offices or on our desks that most of us put in a box and transferred ourselves.

As I was living near the new office at the time of the move, I had all my stuff packed up by early afternoon on the designated Friday and decided to drive over to the new building to see my new office, bringing my little box of personal items with me. As some other departments and staff had already moved over by the time I got there, the building was busy with our own staff, people from the moving firm and contractors who were still painting, fitting carpets and curtains and putting up shelves in offices yet to be occupied.

I found my new office, which was painted and carpeted and, to my eye, finished and ready for my occupation. So I put my little box of personal items on the windowsill and left it there to sort out after the weekend.

The following Monday morning when I arrived, my office furniture was in place and my filing cabinets and boxes of books were stacked around the room. I began to get things organised, and in due course completed everything to my liking. Eventually all that remained was for me to get my personal items placed on my desk and make it truly my office. I went to my little box which was still on the windowsill and looked in. I was stunned to see that three items were not in it. They were three items that I had acquired on my travels and always sat on my desk. They reminded me of places where I had worked or visited, and of the people I had worked with or met there. There was a little carved wooden owl I had bought in Nepal, a small intricately carved soapstone elephant I purchased in India and, most special of all, a little carved wooden man I had bought in Burma, now called Myanmar. They were unique and they were gone. I was absolutely gutted. I never saw them again but I thought about them often, and whenever I was in a charity or thrift shop I always looked at the bric-a-brac sections in case I spotted them. They were insignificant in terms of value but irreplaceable to me, and I missed them.

Over the past year, what had I lost that was irreplaceable, and what did I miss?

I had lost my husband in the truest sense of the word. While Ralph had been leaving me in that role over the previous few years, I realised at this time he was entirely gone from me as my husband. We were truly now the carer and the cared for. He was usually happy and content in my presence and recognised my name, but I was unsure if he knew I was his wife. Neither did I know any more if he knew that some of the nice ladies, as he called them, who came to see him and who hugged and kissed him when they left were his daughters. I had lost intimacy. Of course, I still hugged and kissed him as usual, but he never put his arm around me or kissed me now. He received, but didn't give affection, intimacy or love.

I had lost that wonderful feeling and reality of being truly half of a couple, and as a consequence, both of us had lost the pleasure of sharing life and love. I could no longer share meaningful time together with Ralph. Birthdays and other special events were unknown to him, and thus only noted and celebrated when I did so. The only time I thought Ralph might experience any sense of being half of a couple with me was when he held my hand and stroked it gently. We didn't talk any more about issues, household expenditure, what we would do or where we would go, or even where we had been. I told him where we were going and what we were doing, and made all the arrangements. There were no shared decisions any more, no arguments or disagreements. The house was silent unless this was interrupted by my voice. I talked to him at mealtimes, asked him questions, made comments as we drove in the car but he rarely responded. I had lost my best friend, my life companion, my soulmate. I missed him. It was a lonely place to be.

I had lost the sense each morning as I woke up of it being a new day. Every day was the same and differed only in the appointments that interspersed our weekly routine, or if there were interruptions caused by his deteriorating health. I had lost spontaneity and surprise in my and our lives.

I was so upset at the loss of those three items from my new office that of course I told everyone. A colleague came to me a few days later with a little parcel and said simply, 'For you.' The parcel contained a little soapstone elephant, an exact copy of the one I had lost. She had been in India that year for a holiday and had obviously visited the same craft shops as I had and had bought, as she described it, a herd of these elephants. I still have it, and while it reminds me of the other two items I lost, it was wonderful to have one returned to me in such a special way.

... and found

So, what had I re-found and what unexpected gifts had I gained in the past year? I had discovered a level of patience I never knew I had. I have always been a somewhat impatient person. Part of the control issues, no doubt, but over the past year I had surprised myself with my increasing ability to go at a slower pace, Ralph's pace, and to have patience beyond what I knew was within my own ability as I worked with and cared for him. For the first years of my retirement and prior to his diagnosis, I know I had been very impatient with Ralph at times. I found it frustrating to have to adjust to the slowness with which he dressed or shaved, the speed at which he walked and just the general extension of the time it took him and us to do anything. I had prayed regularly for patience during those years and, certainly in the past one in particular, God had answered my prayers in a way that I never thought possible.

I had deepened my relationship with a number of individuals in ways that would never have happened without the journey Ralph and I had been on. I had become closer to Ralph's family, particularly Lynda, Gwen and Wilma. Closer to my family, to old and new friends and even to our neighbours and people we regularly interacted with in shops, who came to our home, or whom we met at health appointments. I had discovered that there is so much good in people and in our world if only you have the opportunity to see it, and the past year had provided that opportunity for us both. The unexpected acts of kindness that Ralph and I received and continue to receive are such a wonderful gift and so often come at times when they are needed to give me, in particular, strength and hope to go on – like the neighbours who offered help and support, or the coffee shops that gave Ralph a free coffee when he hadn't been in for a while, the pot of soup that appeared and especially the gift of time for me when individuals came and sat with Ralph to let me go out.

I had found a level of acceptance in my life that was now in one sense quiet and alone, but was never fearful or lonely. I had come to appreciate that the greatest treasure I had with Ralph at this time was time itself. Ralph was still with me and I was with him. I had discovered that love between a husband and wife can survive challenges you would never wish on it. We had overcome so many challenges in the early years of our marriage as we readjusted to a life together. They had strengthened us in ways I didn't fully appreciate at the time, but were a reservoir from which we were now able to draw. I was learning that for Ralph and me, love was not fixed but fluid. It may have varied in its expression as it was tried and tested over the past years of his failing health, but love remained. Not pity, not empathy, not affection, but deep love reciprocated in new and different ways, not always obvious but always there, if you only took the time to look for it.

Ralph once told me something his grandmother said: if you were in a group of people who each put their troubles on a table where everyone else could see them, when you saw what everyone else had to bear, you would always take your own troubles home with you. I think there is a great element of truth in that. To some, perhaps his duet of dementia conditions was a trouble they wouldn't want. But I knew that we could bear it because it was our burden – Ralph's, mine and God's – and between the three of us, we could and would cope.

Travelling on together

In my quiet times with God, as well as my daily readings, I always read a few chapters of the Bible without commentary, and at this time I was in the book of Psalms, always a favoured portion. I read again, 'My times are in your hands' (Psalm 31:15). As I reflected on those words, I thought how blessed I was to have my times in God's hands, as they couldn't be in a better place. I certainly wouldn't want them to be in my own hands, as I couldn't cope with that. If I were mistress of my own destiny, goodness knows where I would end up.

Over the year since Ralph's 'D' diagnosis I had come to a total acceptance of the truth of those ancient words, that our times, his and mine, were in God's hands, and I was completely content to leave them there. I had no idea of what the future held and, quite frankly, I didn't want to know. The obsession that some people have with trying to foresee or foretell the future was always lost on me. I have always felt I had quite enough to cope with from day to day without worrying about what might be coming my way in the weeks or months ahead. All I needed to know was that God had our times in His hands, under control and underway in the path that He had determined before we were even born that we should follow. That was sufficient, sure and reassuring.

As Ralph and I moved into our second year of this 'D' journey, in the balancing of the scales between gained and lost, found and gone, enjoyed or missed, I reflected on how we had managed so far. I think we had managed well. Of course, in the past year there had been good times and not-so-good times. There were ups and downs, but we had survived them all, and through them I had gained and learned so much to help me move forward into the next period of our lives. I had learned that I was not alone and that I was surrounded by people and services who were there to help me. I had learned that in the quietness that was now my life, there was a peace and contentment I never would have thought possible as I set off on this journey a year earlier. Despite the challenge that was Ralph's dementia, I had gained a deeper understanding of the man I had married and of myself, and that had brought us a closeness that was special and precious.

As I looked to the second year of our journey, I resolved to look at it as a *plus* one, not a *minus* one. Not one year nearer an end, whatever definition of end I might choose, but rather that it was a gift of a new year for us, a bonus, a plus. Like everyone else setting off on a new year after a particular anniversary, Ralph and I would set off not knowing what it would bring, but with a hope and belief that it would bring us new opportunities and new joys. Whatever challenges we would inevitably meet along the way, I had to believe that they would be overcome and met by and through God's grace.

Again, some words from the Psalms seemed to sum up where I was at this time, one year on, and where Ralph and I were going:

> You make known to me the path of life;
> you will fill me with joy in your presence,
> with eternal pleasures at your right hand.
> *Psalm 16:11*

God didn't only know the path that Ralph and I were travelling on, He also knew where it was taking us, and He would give us joy and delight, both in the travelling along it and in the arrival at our eternal destination. What more could we hope for?

And what about that giant? Where was he? Well, he had reared his ugly head and got behind me a few times over the past year and tried to pull me down. However, by God's grace as I had experienced it through His Word, His children and through the help and support I had received from so many individuals and services, the giant that had crept up behind me and haunted me at times during our 'D' journey over the past year was now where I could see and face him. As we began the second year of our 'D' journey, I knew with certainty that God was bigger than the giant I feared. The proof was that Ralph and I were together, if not more together, one year on from his dementia diagnosis. The journey was to be continued and we would walk on together. Ralph, me and God.

Resources

Everyone who receives a diagnosis of dementia and those who have to share the living out of that diagnosis with them will have different experiences of the disease and its impact. I therefore hesitate to suggest any resources that might prove of help to others, but will humbly share some resources that I have found useful.

www.dementiauk.org
As Ralph was diagnosed with mixed dementia, which is a combination of both Alzheimer's disease and vascular dementia (caused by problems with blood supply to the brain), I found this website particularly helpful. It is easy to navigate and has a wealth of information on all aspects of the diseases in the dementia range, as well as practical advice and details of support for individuals with the diagnosis and their carers.

www.alzheimers.org.uk
This is an easy-to-navigate, very informative website that I went to regularly to check out new information. I particularly liked its research section.

John Dunlop, *Finding Grace in the Face of Dementia* (Wheaton, IL: Crossway, 2017)
I highly recommend this wonderful book written by an American geriatrician with personal experience of dementia in his own family. It includes sections that offer helpful advice for carers, and also a chapter that will challenge churches to reflect on what they could do to support those in their congregations with the disease and those who care for them.

Robin Thomson, *Living with Alzheimer's: A Love Story* (Watford: Instant Apostle, 2020)
This book was published recently so I did not read it during our 'D' journey, but I would recommend it to anyone starting out on a similar journey. Many of the experiences of the writer, as he cared for his wife who had Alzheimer's disease, will resonate with all spouses who care for their loved one through the course of a degenerative condition.

Rosemary Hurtley, *Insight into Dementia*, Waverley Abbey Insight Series (Surrey: CWR, 2013)
A helpful and practical guide for people living with dementia and their carers and families, with suggested activities, reflections and prayers.

Acknowledgements

Writing this first book has been both cathartic and humbling. I am truly indebted to so many people who, when I had the courage to share my first scribbling thoughts with them, gave me so much support and encouragement both to continue writing about this 'D' journey and to endeavour to share it with others.

In particular I want to thank my sister, Liz, who was the first person to read an early draft of this book and who gave me so much encouragement and affirmation in what I had written, which in turn gave me the courage to continue to write. I also want to thank my friend Shirley, who was equally supportive of both my writing and of sharing it with a wider readership.

Ralph's three daughters Lynda, Gwen and Wilma have been my rocks during this year, and their help and support for Ralph and me has been unstinting and so valued and appreciated by us both. I am grateful to all his children for being supportive of this most private man's life at such a difficult time being shared with others through this book.

I am thankful for all of Ralph's and my family's support for us during the year following Ralph's diagnosis. Thank you all for being there with him and with me during some very challenging times.

Thank you to other friends for their encouragement and support, especially Alison, whose reaction to reading an early draft of the book humbled me and confirmed that I should share our 'D' journey with a wider audience.

A special thanks to Kenneth and Mary, our church visitors, but more than that, our friends. Ralph and I always looked forward to your visits with us in our home, and your helpful comments on a draft of this book were greatly appreciated.

My thanks also to Judith for reviewing the book and being supportive of it being shared.

A particular thanks must also go to all the team at Instant Apostle for their guidance, support and patience with me, as we have worked together throughout the publication process.

But most of all I want to thank Ralph. He was and will always be the love of my life.